A Johns Hopkins Press Health Book

The Back Book

Ziya L. Gokaslan, M.D.

Lee Hunter Riley III, M.D.

Illustrated by Ian Suk, B.Sc., B.M.C.

The Johns Hopkins University Press • Baltimore

Note to the Reader

This book is not meant to substitute for the medical care of people with back problems, and treatment should not be based solely on its contents. This book embodies our approach to back problems in general. While we believe and practice its philosophy, we adjust our approach to suit each patient's particular medical condition and situation. We would not treat your back without first learning a great deal about you, and so your treatment should not be based solely on what is written here. It must be developed in a dialogue between you and your physician. Our book is written to help you with that dialogue.

Drug dosage: The authors and publisher have made reasonable efforts to determine that the selection and dosage of drugs discussed in this text conform to the practices of the general medical community. The medications described do not necessarily have specific approval by the U.S. Food and Drug Administration for use in the diseases and dosages for which they are recommended. In view of ongoing research, changes in governmental regulations, and the constant flow of information relating to drug therapy and drug reactions, the reader is urged to check the package insert of each drug for any change in indications and dosage and for warnings and precautions. This is particularly important when the recommended agent is a new and/or infrequently used drug.

© 2008 The Johns Hopkins University Press
Illustrations © 2008 Ian Suk
All rights reserved. Published 2008
Printed in the United States of America on acid-free paper
9 8 7 6 5 4 3 2 1

The Johns Hopkins University Press
2715 North Charles Street
Baltimore, Maryland 21218-4363
www.press.jhu.edu

Library of Congress Cataloging-in-Publication Data

Gokaslan, Ziya L.
The back book / Ziya L. Gokaslan, Lee Hunter Riley III; illustrated by Ian Suk.
    p. cm.
Includes index.
ISBN-13: 978-0-8018-9042-0 (hardcover : alk. paper)
ISBN-10: 0-8018-9042-X (hardcover : alk. paper)
ISBN-13: 978-0-8018-9043-7 (pbk. : alk. paper)
ISBN-10: 0-8018-9043-8 (pbk. : alk. paper)
    1. Backache—Popular works. 2. Backache—Treatment—Popular works. I. Riley, Lee Hunter,
    1960–   . II. Title.
RD771.B217G65 2008
617.5'64   dc22   2008007634

A catalog record for this book is available from the British Library.

Special discounts are available for bulk purchases of this book. For more information, please contact Special Sales at 410-516-6936 or specialsales@press.jhu.edu.

The Johns Hopkins University Press uses environmentally friendly book materials, including recycled text paper that is composed of at least 30 percent post-consumer waste, whenever possible. All of our book papers are acid-free, and our jackets and covers are printed on paper with recycled content.

Contents

Illustrations appear following page 70

The Back Book

Introduction
As Common as the Common Cold and Twenty Times More Painful

WE TALK TO MANY people with back pain, both to individual patients and to groups. When we are invited to speak to a group of people who are interested in back problems, we ask the audience, "How many people here have ever had the common cold?" And *every person in the room raises their hand.* Then we ask, "How many people go to the doctor when they get a cold?" *Nobody raises their hand.*

We then ask, "How many people have had back pain?" Again, *everybody raises their hand.*

"Who went to the doctor the first time they had back pain?" *Everybody raises their hand.*

"Who went to the doctor the second or third time they had back pain?" *And a lot of people raise their hand.*

The purpose of this book is to explore the reasons for back pain and when and why you should see a doctor, if at all. When you consider how common back pain is—80 percent of Americans will suffer back pain at some point in their lives—you see why these questions about the common cold are relevant. Like the common cold, back pain is common. And also like a cold, back pain generally goes away on its own, without treatment of any kind other than comfort measures. But episodes of back pain are not frequent enough that you can develop an understanding of the problem and the natural history of it, the same way you do with a cold. One of the reasons people are more likely to seek help for back pain is that the pattern is not immediately recognizable because it is not as frequent—you do not get it every winter or every other winter, as you do a cold. Another reason is that back pain can be so very painful and uncomfortable and can keep you from living your life normally.

In general, you do not need to be treated by a doctor for back pain because the pain usually goes away in a couple of days to a couple of weeks (although it could go on for several months). Even if pain lasts up to two months, you still do not need to have an x-ray. At most, you may need your internist or family doctor to perform a physical examination and record your medical history. However, you will want to ensure that back pain is not the result of a more serious problem. *You need to see a doctor sooner than two months after the pain begins if any of the following apply to you:*

- If the pain is incapacitating.
- If you have a history of cancer and back pain occurs for no reason.
- If the pain is constant.
- If the pain wakes you up at night or if you are in constant pain that keeps you awake.
- If you have fever, chills, weight loss, or have had a recent infection.
- If you have cancer.
- If you fell or suffered trauma that caused back pain.
- If you have leg pain below your knees.
- If you notice any change in bowel or bladder function.
- If you feel any numbness, tingling, or weakness.

Doctors divide back pain into two general categories—acute and chronic. Acute back pain lasts less than six months (most often much less) and is the most common type experienced. Chronic back pain lasts more than six months, is less common than acute back pain, but its cost to society in lost wages and medical expenses is much greater than acute back pain.

Here is our prescription for moderate, garden-variety acute back pain with no accompanying weakness or paralysis:

- Initially, treat with short-term bed rest for a day or two.
- Take anti-inflammatory medications right away to reduce the inflammation in the muscles, joints, and discs, which is a common cause of back pain. Expect to take these medications regularly for up to two weeks before they have their full effect.
- Gradually increase your activities.
- Take a muscle relaxant if prescribed by your physician for a couple of days or up to one week if you have painful and frequent back spasms and only if needed.

A short course of narcotic pain medication can be used for extreme pain to enable people to resume their activities or gain mobility. Narcotic medication will not eliminate pain but can take the edge off the pain so you can move around: *The key to getting better with back pain is to get up and resume normal activities as soon as possible.* We cannot overemphasize the role of activity in recovering from back pain.

Chronic back pain is continuous back pain that lasts greater than six months. Unless there is a clear, specific reason for chronic back pain, surgery is not recommended. An operation can worsen chronic back pain, which is, for most people, a nonsurgical condition.

When the cause of pain can be identified in the small number of people with chronic back pain, surgery can reduce or eliminate the pain. This group is much smaller than the group that does not benefit from surgery, however. For most people, nonsurgical options are recommended and are successful in treating back pain.

What about Back Surgery?

The source of back pain is often difficult or impossible to identify. This can be frustrating to patients who know they have pain but cannot be given a specific reason they are experiencing the pain. It can be difficult for the person experiencing pain and for others (friends, family, and colleagues) to understand why the pain is happening without a specific cause.

Despite our best efforts to identify the cause of back pain, a specific cause is often not discovered by the medical community. This does not mean that a person does not have pain or that the pain cannot be treated. Treatment needs to be tailored to the specific person and the cause of the pain. Treatment can range from exercises and medications to surgery. In Chapter 8, we discuss why someone might have surgery. Having good reasons to have surgery and rational expectations for the results of surgery is crucial. Even with advice from many sources, each person has to decide whether to have surgery. Some people want to continue functioning at their current level, and because their quality of life is deteriorating, they choose surgery. Some people with spinal stenosis, for example, have surgery when standing or walking is difficult.

Recovery and improvement vary depending on the operation. For example, someone who has surgery to treat sciatica from the lumbar disc may wake up in the recovery room feeling better than before the surgery. For other conditions, a patient may begin to feel better soon after the surgery, but the full benefits from the operation are not apparent for three, six, or up to twelve months. The extent and difficulty of the operation and the age of the person also affect the pace of recovery. We discuss all of these issues in later chapters.

About This Book

Back conditions can be crippling, can pose many questions, and can offer few answers. In *The Back Book*, we strive to provide a balanced overview of options for the millions of people suffering with problems with their back. Our six major goals in writing the book follow:

1. To help the person with a back problem develop reasonable expectations concerning the condition, and to avoid disappointment with its treatment.
2. To establish that each back condition requires individualized treatment.
3. To explain why and how the physician or surgeon and patient should arrive at a treatment plan that is acceptable to both.

4. To explain why back pain and surgery can be so complicated.
5. To explain back surgery so readers understand the possibilities it offers as well as its risks and limitations.
6. To explain how to choose a surgeon as well as how to choose the right surgeon.

Because of the many different approaches to treating the spine, patients need to be informed about and actively participate in their care decisions. In this book, readers will gain a better understanding of the anatomy of their back, the multiple causes of back problems, the diagnostic process, and the treatment options available, including some promising new technologies. By explaining that realistic goals often result in better outcomes, we hope to reassure readers that, while problems with your back cannot always be cured, it is often possible to minimize pain and improve the quality of life.

Finally, despite everything we do to try to diagnose, to identify, and to treat patients' pain, there are still patients whose pain will not be eliminated or function improved. We will not be able to find out exactly what's wrong with every patient, and despite our best efforts with medical treatment and sometimes surgery, some patients will still have a lot of pain. For them, chronic pain management generally provides some relief.

In Part I, we examine some of the many conditions, disorders, and events that may lead to back pain. In Part II, we describe approaches to treating pain, including medical treatment, physical therapy, surgery, and management of chronic pain.

Part I
What's Causing Your Symptoms?

One
Twenty-Four Vertebrae and Twenty-Three Discs

IN THIS CHAPTER WE provide a short refresher course in the anatomy of the spine to explain what's going on in your back (and in the rest of this book). We conclude with the lower back because that is where most back problems occur.

Back problems are common because modern humans live longer, and joints and other body parts wear out as they age. It may be comforting (although it won't lessen your pain) to know that most back problems are a lot like getting gray hair: They are a normal part of the aging process.

The Five Regions of the Spine

The *spinal column* is composed of bones and discs, the *muscles* and *ligaments* that support the bones and discs, and the *spinal cord* and *nerves*, all of which work together to allow us to move—to turn our neck, to bend over, to twist, and to sit. The *vertebral column* is made up of the vertebrae (the backbones). The vertebral column protects and channels all the nerves in the body. The spinal *cord* is the main part of the nervous system through which all the nerves in the body travel, sending signals back and forth from the brain and the body (see Figure 1). Muscles and ligaments provide stability and support for the other structures. We move when our muscles respond to signals sent by the nerves.

The spine is divided into five primary regions: (1) the *cervical spine* (the neck), (2) the *thoracic spine* (the chest region, or the middle of the back), (3) the *lumbar spine* (the lower back), (4) the *sacrum* (a specialized part of the spinal column consisting of vertebrae that are fused together into one bone that forms part of the pelvis), and (5) the *coccyx* (a rudimentary tail with little functional significance). The first four regions play an important role in supporting the body and positioning it in space. The cervical spine supports the head and helps control the arms. The neck generally moves freely, from side to side and backward and forward. Because the thoracic spine attaches to the ribs, which prevent the body from bending to the side, motion in that region of the spine is mostly rotation. The anatomy in the lumbar region allows for a lot of movement: forward, backward, and to the side. Below the lumbar region of the spine fused vertebrae form a triangular bone called the *sacrum*, and below the sacrum is the very small "tail" bone called the *coccyx*. The sacrum is one of the bones that form the pelvis (see Figure 2).

The cervical spine, thoracic spine, lumbar spine, and sacrum provide the four curves in the back. These curves are the normal bends in the back that you can see by looking at yourself sideways in a full-length mirror. They help us with balance, flexibility, and stress absorption. If they need to, the curves can collapse like an accordion to absorb shocks. The four curves are

1. cervical lordosis (*lordosis* here simply means a backward bend);
2. thoracic kyphosis (*kyphosis* means a forward bend);
3. lumbar lordosis (another backward bend); and
4. sacral curve kyphosis (another forward bend).

Lordosis means the back bends toward the back of the body, forming a **C** shape; *kyphosis* means the back bends toward the front of the body (see Figure 2). Some conditions in the back, such as scoliosis, cause an exaggeration or flattening of these (see Chapter 3).

The Bones and the Joints

Bone is an active organ of the body made up of collagen, minerals, proteins, and living cells. It is continually manufactured and broken down. To manufacture bone properly, critical components must be in place and activated. Building blocks such as vitamin D and calcium must be available to make bone. Cells (osteoblasts, osteoclasts, and osteocytes), hormones, and signaling proteins play roles in the formation of bone. Any deficiencies or imbalance in these factors can cause changes in bone formation, leading to imperfect and weakened bone.

If we do not form adequate bones as children, we may very well have weak bones as adults. Physical activity (walking, running, jumping, and other sports) and taking vitamins and calcium supplements early in life significantly affect how strong bones are going to be as you age. If children's calcium intake is not adequate, they do not receive enough vitamin D, or the vitamins are not activated, then they will not have strong bones as adults.

The bones in the back support the rest of the body, allow for movement, and protect the spinal cord. Most people are familiar with the vertebrae and discs in the back, but there are also other bones.

The Vertebrae

The vertebrae are stacked atop one another and are connected together with vertebral discs and facet joints. Beginning at the base of the skull and moving down, the cervical spine consists of the first seven vertebrae, the thoracic spine consists of the next twelve vertebrae, and the lumbar spine consists of the bottom five vertebrae. Five fused sacral vertebrae form the triangular-shaped sacral bone that is the posterior part of the pelvis. Below the sacrum are four coccygeal segments that are the vestiges of a rudimentary tail. The vertebrae are numbered C1 through C7, T1 through T12, and L1 through L5, and. Numbering always begins at the top of the region. Thus, C1 is the vertebra located just below the skull, T1 begins just below C7, and L1 is located below T12 (see Figure 3). These important markers are used in describing the location of a back problem. Your doctor may tell you that you have a disc bulging in the L4-5 area, for example. The vertebrae are the big, bony building blocks of the spine. The vertebrae in each of the three regions of the spine are different sizes. The neck bones are relatively small and allow the neck to move freely, whereas the lumbar vertebrae are large and thick. Regardless of their size, all vertebrae have the same parts (see Figure 4). The front of each vertebra is called the *vertebral body*. The other parts are the pedicle, the transverse process, the lamina, and the spinous process. The vertebral foramen is the opening where the nerves exit the spinal canal.

- The vertebral body is the big part of the bone.
- The pedicle is the column of bone that connects the vertebral body in front to the posterior element in the back. Each vertebra has two pedicles.
- The lamina form the roof over the spinal canal.
- The facet is the point through which adjacent vertebrae articulate.
- The pars interarticularis is the narrow bridge of bone joining the lamina and inferior articular facet to the pedicle and superior facet.

The Discs and the Facet Joints

Each pair of vertebrae is connected in the front with a disc and in the back with two *facet joints*. One intervertebral disc connects each pair of vertebrae in the front of the spinal column, and a pair of joints connects each pair in the back. Thus, there are essentially three joints: the disc in front and two facet joints in back. Like the joints in the knee or the hip, the joints in the spine bend and rotate to make it possible for us to move.

The discs are located between the vertebral bodies and function as shock absorbers. A disc is a very specialized joint—it's a joint because it moves, but it doesn't move as much as joints in other parts of the body (like the knee). This specialized joint serves two functions:

1. It transmits forces up and down the body and spreads the load out evenly from one joint to the next.
2. It allows us to twist, to rotate, and to bend.

Two specialized components of the disc give it the ability to spread loads or forces out across the bone evenly and allow motion. One of these components is the center of the disc, called the *nucleus pulposus*, which is composed of jelly-like cartilage with a lot of water in it. The other component is a tough, rubbery portion of the disc called the *annulus fibrosis*, which goes around the nucleus pulposis to hold in the jelly-like substance of the nucleus pulposis. This outer rim is made up of layers of cartilage arranged like the steel belts of a radial tire (see Figure 5).

The other joints are called the facet joints; they are the connections between the bones. The inferior facet articulates with, or is jointed with, the superior facet of the vertebra below, and the superior facet articulates with the inferior facet of the vertebra above.

Unlike the discs, the facet joints are classic joints, similar to your elbow, your knee, or your hip. Hip, knee, and facet joints, are *synovial joints* because they are surrounded by *synovium*, a specialized inner layer or lining of the joint that creates a lubricant called *synovial fluid*, which is like oil. The synovium creates synovial fluid and fills the joint with it.

Each pair of facets on either side of the vertebrae connects the vertebrae to the vertebra above and below forming a facet joint. The facet joints are composed of *articular cartilage, synovial fluid* (that fluid lubricant), and a *joint capsule*. Articular cartilage means "joint cartilage"; it is the surface of the joint, and it helps support the joint and allows it to move. Synovial fluid is a lubricant for the cartilage that allows the cartilage to glide without much friction. The facet joint capsules can be thought of as the "gristle"—the rubbery, elastic structures that form the outer layer of the joints. All joints with articular cartilage and synovial fluid have a capsule as their outer layer.

When we're young, these structures in the back are nice and healthy. As we age, however, they stiffen up and become thickened or calcified, and then a whole set of problems arises. As the facet joint becomes arthritic, the cartilage wears out and thins out, and the underlying bone is exposed. The body reacts by limiting the motion of the joint, creating bone spurs, and doing other things that enlarge the joint. In other words, aging affects joints by making them bigger. As joints get bigger, they take up more space in the spinal canal, which makes the canal narrower and causes problems such as spinal stenosis, a narrowing of the spinal canal.

The Sacrum and the Coccyx

At the bottom of the last vertebra in the lumbar region of the spine, all the sacral vertebrae are fused together to form the triangular structure known as the *sacrum*. The sacrum is attached on either side to the iliac bones, which contain the socket portion of the ball-and-socket hip joint. Together the sacrum and iliac bones form the pelvis. At the bottom of the sacrum is the coccyx, our rudimentary tail, or tailbone, where the sacrum and the iliac join at the sacroiliac joint. The first sacral vertebra is labeled S1.

Muscles and Ligaments

Outside these structures are various ligaments and muscles attached to the spinal column. A *ligament* is a band of tissue that connects bones or supports internal organs. The ligaments in the back are thick, rubbery elastic structures that stretch when you bend but also provide structural support for the bones (see Figure 5). If they are torn or injured, ligaments can become sore.

Muscles produce movement by contracting in response to signals from the nerves. The *abdominal muscles* help stabilize the spine and connect the ribs down to the pelvis. The large muscles that attach across the back are called *paraspinus muscles*. They are connected to the transverse processes and spinous process of the vertebral body. The *psoas muscle*, located in the front of the lumbar spine, is connected to the spine, runs down to the thigh, and allows the hip to bend.

Muscles can be bruised or torn in a variety of ways including in a sports injury or a car crash, or even in a slip on the ice or raking leaves. Keeping muscles toned and maintained helps enormously with back health. If there is weakness in or injury to abdominal or paraspinus muscles or the psoas muscle, joints and other muscles in the spine will be stressed and may become a source of pain.

We (and most other doctors) believe that the most important back muscles are the abdominal muscles because strong abdominal muscles provide strong support for the structures in the back, keeping them aligned to maintain a healthy posture. A person with good posture and a well-supported back will have an easier time avoiding back problems. (We discuss important strengthening exercises in Chapter 7.)

The Spinal Cord and Nerves

The *spinal canal* is the main tunnel in the vertebrae through which all the nerves run. It is an oval- or round-shaped space covered with a membrane called the *dura*. The spinal canal contains the spinal cord and the nerves that come out of the spinal cord and travel to the lower extremities. At each vertebrae, a pair of nerves exit out to the rest of the body, one nerve going to the right side and one to the left side. The nerves exit next to the joints, through a structure called the *foramen* (pronounced "for-A-men"; *foramen* in Latin means "hole").

The spinal cord is divided into the same four regions as the spinal column. Each region of the spinal cord helps to control different functions. The cervical spinal cord contributes to function in the neck and arms; the thoracic region controls muscles in the chest that help with breathing and coughing; and the lumbrosacral spinal cord helps control the legs, pelvis, bowel, and bladder.

Different kinds of nerves in the body serve different functions. Sensory nerves carry signals to the brain from the skin ("I'm cold!") and outer structures of the body as well as from structures deep inside the body ("My back is killing me!"). The motor nerves also carry signals from the brain to the body, to move muscles and control movement. The autonomic nerves keep the body functioning automatically. They control heart rate, blood flow, and digestion—all of the so-called involuntary process over which we consciously have little or no control.

The spinal cord, which is like an electrical cable that carries all the signals both ways between the brain and the body, is a compact tubular structure that goes all the way down to the L1 or L2 level. The nerves come out all along the cable (through the foramen). When the spinal cord is healthy, round, and "free" and the nerves are not impinged, signals travel unimpaired between the body and the brain. When the spinal cord or a nerve becomes pinched for any reason, however, the signals are interrupted, communication breaks down, and function can be impaired. The range of problems that can develop is wide: a person can have trouble walking or may have difficulty with bladder or bowel control. Impingement of the nerve or spinal cord is a frequent source of pain, as well. The spinal cord is a delicate structure, whereas the nerves are more resistant to pressure or to damage and are able to recover their function more easily than the spinal cord. Figure 1 shows the spinal cord in relation to the vertebrae and nerves, including the sciatic nerve (see Chapter 3).

That Essential—and Problematic—Lumbar Region

The thoracic region is well supported and has limited motion. Because it does not move much, it is seldom a source of pain related to wear and tear on the joints. The cervical spine can be the source of pain. Nerve compression in the neck causes pain in the arm rather than in the leg and it can also interfere with sexual function and function of the bowel and bladder.

We primarily focus on the lumbar region because when someone has a back problem, the lumbar spine is generally the source of the problem. For one thing, the body's weight is transmitted through the lumbar spine to the pelvis and then to the legs down to the ground. Also the lumbar spine is a flexible structure; it moves in different directions, and it twists around. It acts as a series of joints so that the upper torso can be positioned in space with respect to the legs. Finally, at the L1 or L2 level, called the *cauda equina,* or horse's tail, all the nerves come out, resembling hairs of the horse's tail.

The spine serves a couple of functions. First, it acts as a channel, or conduit, and a protector for all the nerves in the body before they branch out and go down the arms and legs and to other parts of your body. Second, it functions as a series of joints connected together that allows positioning of the body in space. It allows us to bend over, to move, to twist.

Some of the problems we will address in this book relate to how the structures in the lumbar spine fail to function as a series of joints or fail to function as the conduit for the nerves (fail to provide enough space for the nerves to travel through). Arthritis, for example, affects joints all over the body. In the spine, it can cause a disc to slip or herniate and can also cause spinal stenosis, which is a narrowing of the tunnel where the nerve runs. Figures 6 and 7 illustrate some common causes of back pain; these conditions are described in the next two chapters.

As we have seen, the anatomy of the back is complex. In fact, many people are surprised by the back's numerous functions and how many structures there are in the back. It's no wonder, really, that so much can go wrong in the back. In the next chapter, we begin to explore some of these issues.

Two

Who Gets Back Pain, and What Causes It?

NEARLY EVERYONE HAS BACK pain at some time in his or her life. The pain might come on intensely and suddenly, when they twist to catch a long pass in a backyard football game, or it might come on gradually and settle in, which is what happens to many people as they get older. It only makes sense that people who play hard or work hard physically are more likely to develop back pain. But a sedentary lifestyle is also bad for the back. Genetics can play a role in determining who develops a back condition that causes pain, and diet and other factors also influence the health of the back.

Because so many people have back pain, it may seem that just being human can cause back pain. That's not far from the truth because sitting and walking upright, as humans do, puts enormous stress on the back. As noted previously, back pain is as prevalent as the common cold. Moreover, most back pain is as benign as the common cold. But since back pain doesn't happen on a recurring basis (like a cold), people are more likely to seek medical attention for it. If you experience back pain after raking leaves or lifting a heavy box, and if your back pain doesn't include sciatica (leg weakness, pain, numbness, or tingling), then you are joining a very large group of people: over the course of their lives, most people will develop that kind of back pain. More than half of them will have pain severe enough to take time off from work.

Every single nerve in our body has a function: Motor nerves serve a motor function (movement), and sensory nerves serve a sensation function (feeling). Pain is the protective sensation that makes us pull our hand away automatically if we touch a hot stove. Pain alerts us when something is wrong in our body. When the motor function of a nerve is impaired, it impairs a certain set of muscles that have a certain function. When sensation is compromised, it leads to a loss or alteration of sensation in a specific area.

Nerve irritation can be caused by chemical irritation, like a bee sting, and mechanical pressure, like having an eyelash in your eye or getting your toe stepped on. Take a ruptured (herniated) disc, for example (discussed in Chapter 3). The nerve is directly pushed by the disc material causing a mechanical irritation, but there's also inflammation (the chemical reaction) that occurs when the disc material spills into the epidural space. The combined mechanical irritation and chemical irritation of the nerve leads to pain. The chemical irritation also makes the nerve more sensitive to any mechanical pressure. In its sensitive state, if you apply any kind of mechanical pressure or stimulation to the nerve, that extra stimulus causes more symptoms.

Some people can tolerate a lot of pain and other people can tolerate very little pain. There is no way to objectively scale pain and grade it from one person to the next, which is why pain is a difficult symptom to treat. It is a subjective symptom. When someone has leg numbness or leg weakness, the degree of numbness or weakness can be assessed: We can tell whether their strength has improved or the sensation has improved in their leg, but we can't really assess the degree of pain—we can't tell how *bad* it is.

We've already seen how complicated a structure the back is, and it's easy to understand how things can go wrong when there are so many moving parts. In the next chapter, we'll explore the specific conditions that cause back pain, including some conditions that aren't located in the back. In this chapter, we take a bird's-eye view of the causes of back pain and who is most likely to have back pain.

The Aging Spine

With increased age the likelihood of developing health problems of all kinds increases. A person whose muscles have become weaker or whose bones have become somewhat brittle is more likely to be injured, and a disease process that has been developing over time can "announce itself" in the older person.

Some people define aging as losing flexibility, and if you think about it, it is often easy to tell whether someone is old or young by the way they walk. An older person often doesn't have the same bounce as a young person. As the body ages, the structures in the back age, too. They are not as flexible as they once were, and they start to wear out.

To put things into perspective: If anything narrows the space where the nerves are traveling, that narrowed space puts pressure on the nerve, and that pressure can create a whole set of problems, including pain, numbness, weakness, and problems with function. For example, if a disc ages and begins to bulge into the spinal canal, there is narrowing of the space where the nerves travel, which can lead to pressure on the nerves. To take another example, if the ligaments and the joints thicken, that thickening also narrows the space where the nerves are traveling. Or if one vertebra slips with respect to the other one, that makes the space narrower.

Arthritis

Arthritis is a normal part of the aging process (though that doesn't mean we have to like it). One form is *degenerative arthritis*, which is the result of joints essentially wearing over time. It happens in various parts of the body: in the joints in your hands, your wrists, your hip, your ankle, your knee, your shoulder—all of these large joints can be affected by arthritis, the wear and tear that occurs over time as a result of repeated use. A person with arthritis usually wakes up in the morning stiff and uncomfortable and then, as he or she moves around, the person loosens up. At the end of day, however, the pain usually returns because the person will have repeatedly used the worn-out joint.

The articular cartilage inside the joint that functions as a cushion wears out, and then the surrounding bone becomes inflamed and causes pain. Similar processes happen in the spine as well. We talked earlier about the joints behind the facet joints, which are small gliding surfaces. As a person ages, over time the disc space collapses, the joints become worn out, and the person can have pain similar to the pain arthritis causes in other joints. The discs also wear out, narrow, and bulge.

Arthritis in the back can trigger muscle spasms in the back, mimicking typical lumbar sprain or disc herniation. The pain can also radiate down to the buttocks and the upper part of the leg but not generally all the way down to the back of the leg, to the calf or foot, as we commonly see with herniated disc or lumbar stenosis or any condition of the nerve that contributes to sciatica.

In the diagnosis of arthritis in the spine, we obtain plain x-ray studies, which can demonstrate the worn-out joints. A computed tomography (CT) scan of the lumbar joints is particularly helpful because it gives us a fairly good detail of the bony structures of these joints. A magnetic resonance imaging (MRI) scan can also be done to illustrate how the nerves that travel through that area are affected by arthritis.

Because it is common to see facet joint wear on x-ray studies, and because most people with these x-ray findings do not have symptoms, we cannot assume that facet joint wear is the cause of the pain. We have to rely on other methods of diagnosis to ensure that the arthritic facet joint is causing pain. The *facet block* test is done by introducing a needle through the back to the region of these joints. We inject a local anesthetic mixed with steroids into the facet joint so that the nerves that carry the pain signals from these joints can be blocked. If the pain decreases, we can then be reasonably confident that the facet abnormalities that we see on the x-ray studies are responsible for your pain. (Facet block is described in Chapters 5 and 6.)

If the usual conservative measures that we take in treating any back condition (see Chapter 6) are unsuccessful, a treatment of this condition can be a procedure called a *facet radiofrequency denervation* (*denervation* means "to remove the nerve"). It is done similarly to the facet block, but this time the probe is introduced close to the specific nerves that carry the pain signals from the facet joints. The nerves are burned using a radiofrequency signal to heat up the tip of the needle. This procedure can be successful in alleviating pain, but it may not permanently relieve the discomfort—the pain may return after six months or a year. Repeated or subsequent facet radiofrequency denervation procedures are not as successful. There is not a good surgical solution for facet-related problems. As a last resort, a fusion can be performed, which eliminates the motion in that joint; however, the success of the surgery is limited. In one study to determine whether patients with a positive facet block test improved if they were treated with a fusion procedure, the results did not indicate whether a fusion is helpful in these circumstances. Either our operation is not exactly directed at the pathology or our diagnostic testing is not adequate to tell us where the pain is coming from.

Degenerative arthritis is degenerative joint disease just as we see anywhere else in the body. Some individuals, however, have arthritic conditions such as rheumatoid arthritis (RA); systemic lupus erythematosus (a chronic inflammatory disorder of connective tissue); or other rheumatological conditions that can cause inflammation of the synovial joints (the joints that contain fluid) as well as facet joints. These joints can become inflamed and are eventually destroyed by the disease process. Destruction of the joints can cause pain similar to the pain we see with degenerative arthritis, but it is much more severe and affects many joints and not just in one area, whereas degenerative arthritis tends to affect the joints that are most under stress. Those arthritic conditions need to be treated medically with drugs aimed at minimizing the inflammation in the joints. It is unusual for someone to be newly diagnosed with RA or these other conditions because of back pain; usually they have a known history of RA or another condition, or they have typical signs of these arthritic conditions when a neurosurgeon or orthopedic surgeon sees the patient because of back pain.

Osteoporosis

Osteoporosis is another age-related process. Many people don't know that bone is both made and broken down each day. Most people *do* know that the hormone estrogen helps with bone formation and that women produce less estrogen after menopause. Osteoporosis is not just a problem for women, but it is not as common in men because of their greater average bone mass. When someone has osteoporosis, his or her bones become weaker. A well-known manifestation of osteoporosis is hip fractures, which we see in people in their sixties and seventies—more commonly in women than in men. In a similar fashion, the vertebral bodies in the spinal column can fracture. We call these *osteoporotic compression fractures*.

To get a sense of the problem, think about looking inside a bone. The vertebral body is a cylindrical block: there is a top to it, there is a bottom to it, and there are walls. Within that cylindrical block, you have a cage with reinforcing spickles, like the reinforcing iron bars, or rebar, put inside a hollow surface before cement is poured into it. If you cut a bone and look through it, you will see that the spickles are woven.

As osteoporosis sets in, two things occur: (1) the space between rods increases and (2) the rods become thinner. As a result, the block is more prone to collapse under any kind of weight, which is a *compression fracture*. The bone, and particularly the spine, cannot carry the load that is placed on it because the bone has been weakened substantially. (Osteoporosis is like cheating on the iron support system. You and the contractor have agreed that the contractor is going to use sixteen iron bars to support your cement column; as you get older, what happens, is [1] the contractor uses thinner iron bars and [2] he says, "To conserve on the cost, I'm going to space them out." Instead of using sixteen of them, he uses eight. As you can imagine, the column cannot support the same weight. This is what happens with progressive osteoporosis.)

Bone mass is measured using a bone density scan. The numerical value of an individual's bone density is compared with the bone of healthy, young individuals. If the bone density matches the healthy individual—if the score is in the middle of the bell curve—then the value is 0. If the value falls into the first or second set of deviations, a score of 1 or 2 is given. The farther the score is away from 0, the weaker the bone, and the higher the risk of having a significant fracture in the hip, the wrist, or the spinal column. Typically, a 30- or 35-year-old woman will fall into the 0 to 1 range on the bone density measurement. Someone with a score greater than 1.5 standard deviations from 0 has definite osteoporosis that requires treatment. Someone with a score greater than 2.5 standard deviations away from the medium is at substantial risk of fracture. Many studies have looked at the issue of osteoporosis. The key is to find a treatment for osteoporosis that stops or slows the process of degeneration. A number of medications are used to treat osteoporosis. Fosomax, one of the most common medications decreases bone breakdown by specifically inhibiting the cells that do this job in the bone. On this medication, you don't necessarily manufacture more bone, but you don't break it down as fast. As a result, the balance is in favor of bone formation and therefore a reduction in the risk of fracture down the line, and this can be demonstrated visibly on bone densometer measurements. Calcitonin also treats osteoporosis. It is a hormone produced by the parathyroid gland that naturally aids in bone formation. Calcitonin is taken in a nasal spray.

Calcium and vitamin supplements are commonly given to women with osteoporosis to increase their capacity to augment bone, but these supplements are not effective themselves because women's capacity to form bones after a certain age is not good. For that reason, another strategy is to use supplementary estrogen to help with bone formation, but supplementary estrogen (called hormone replacement therapy, or HRT) comes with an increased risk of uterine cancer, and some data indicate that breast cancer chances are also increased.

Osteoporotic vertebral compression fractures can happen in many vertebrae over time. People become more stooped over, or *kyphotic*, because of the fractures. *Kyphosis*, remember, is a forward bend; it creates the "hunchbacked" posture, or "widow's hump," of many older people. Many compression fractures heal on their own and don't pose any major problems, although they heal in a shortened position and the spine loses its normal configuration. More serious problems occur when a vertebral body collapses, causing severe angulation of the spinal column, with bone fragments going into the spinal canal and causing spinal cord compression or nerve compression, weakness or paralysis, or loss of bowel or bladder control. Quality of life suffers greatly. It is much more difficult to deal with these problems, and it can be difficult to get relief from the pain. Although most compression fractures heal with time, with the help of a brace and rest, some of them become intractable in terms of pain, and if the neurological structures are affected and are in turn affecting function, then urgent surgical intervention is needed.

Typically, then, compression fractures of the spine are treated with medications and bracing, and within two to three months, the fracture heals and the patient's pain subsides. If pain remains persistent or severe, then, in addition to pain medications and other symptomatic treatments, we also do either a *vertebroplasty* or a *kyphoplasty*, which involves injecting bone cement into the fractured vertebral body to immediately stabilize the fracture and strengthen the vertebral body. It is injected in a thick liquid consistency and then hardens (see Chapter 6).

Degenerative Disc Disease

Like joints and bones, discs wear out as we age. Different types of degeneration can happen to the disc. When we are young and healthy, the middle portion of the disc is nice and juicy, while the other part is tough and rubbery. As we age, the disc cartilage changes and can lead to disc bulging, herniation, and alteration in the physical properties of discs. (see Chapter 3).

Unhealthy Habits

A lifetime of smoking, a poor diet, or a sedentary lifestyle can easily lead to back pain. We know that smokers have a greater incidence of back pain than nonsmokers. Someone who exercises regularly is less likely to have back pain.

The older we are, the more likely it is that the damaging effects of chronic diseases, such as diabetes, high blood pressure (hypertension), and obesity, will affect our nervous system and circulatory system, possibly resulting in pain in the back and down the legs. In some instances, not only is back pain caused by diseases but also by treatment for the diseases. Bronchial asthma, chronic pulmonary disease, rheumatoid arthritis—all may require high doses of steroids to treat the underlying condition, but long-term steroid use may lead to osteoporosis, which, as we have seen, can lead to compression fractures and pain.

Finally, as time passes, we are more likely to develop a new disease, such as cancer. Back pain can be caused by a tumor in the back, by metastases from breast cancer or prostate cancer, or by cancer that begins elsewhere in the body, and it can be caused by cancer elsewhere that sends pain signals to the back (see Chapter 4).

The Stressed and Injured Spine

Olympic gymnasts twist their bodies to perform seemingly impossible physical feats. Ballet dancers rise up on their toes and then leap through the air. Basketball players charge up and down the floor shooting hoops. Football players throw themselves through the air and land on the ground (or another player). Volleyball players jump and reach to spike the ball over the net. When they are not performing or competing, these artists and entertainers are practicing. It's amazing, when you think about it, that more gymnasts, ballet dancers, and athletes playing impact sports don't wind up with back pain. Many of them do, of course. They stress their backs by hyperextending and may end up with an injury, possibly one that keeps them from performing or playing. They may pull their muscles, tear a ligament, or develop a condition called *spondylolysis*, which is a crack in the pars interarticularis. (Spondylolysis may be acquired early in life or from trauma; it is discussed in Chapter 3.)

Professionals are not the only ones sidelined by back pain. Weekend athletes, older athletes, and athletes whose cardiovascular conditioning doesn't protect their joints from the stress of twisting, running, and jumping, may be sidelined, too. The 40-year-old who played basketball in college and has been working at a desk for twenty years may end up in the doctor's office after a pickup basketball game. And so may the weekend gardener who stretches to pull weeds on a Saturday afternoon.

In the workplace, both the physically active worker and the sedentary worker are at risk for back pain. Lift a box the wrong way and the UPS delivery person is in an agony of back spasm. Strain over a stack of invoices and a computer for hours on end and the accountant stands up, grimacing, holding his lower back. The back can be easily injured. If you stretch, twist, pull, or strain the structures in your back beyond their limits, the structures become irritated and inflamed—and that leads to pain. Muscles can easily be stretched or torn through overexertion or overuse. In fact, muscle strain, and in particular lumbar sprain, is the most common back problem and is usually related to physical activity that stresses the back (see Chapter 3).

Although it is almost certainly the result of an ongoing process, disc degeneration often shows up rather abruptly, as acute, excruciating pain. In other words, the symptoms are usually associated with some kind of physical activity, but the problem has often been brewing for a longer period.

As we noted in Chapter 1, most doctors say that the most important back muscles are the abdominal muscles. This fact is especially relevant during pregnancy when many women feel back pain because their abdominal muscles are stretched out of shape for nine months. Furthermore, during pregnancy the ligaments become soft and loose, and as the baby descends into the pelvis during delivery, the baby puts pressure on the sciatic nerve. Some women develop sciatica (pain in the sciatic nerve) during pregnancy, though it clears up after delivery. After the baby is born, the new mother is likely to have pain from her now out-of-shape muscles as she carries an ever-growing baby around. When she lies down and takes the weight off, the pain goes away.

Disease and the Spine

When a physician examines someone age 50 or older, chronic medical conditions such as diabetes and cancer are special concerns. Anyone who has had recent surgery and an infection will also be a cause for concern. Many kinds of systemic diseases cause back conditions that cause pain, and the physician will want to determine whether the pain is part of an ongoing disease process, the result of normal aging, or an injury.

A person with a systemic disease or a condition elsewhere in the body—such as a tumor or ballooning of the aorta (called an aneurism), kidney stones, or an infection in the abdomen—may have referred pain in the back. (Referred pain means that a problem elsewhere is exciting nerves that send signals to the back, and though the back is not causing the pain, the brain locates and experiences the pain in the back.)

The Genetic Component

We know that there is a genetic component to back pain for some people because clusters of ruptured discs can occur in families. Eskimos, for example, are known to have a genetic predisposition for back problems. In addition, some collagen vascular diseases, such as Marfan syndrome and Ehlers-Danlos syndrome, affect all kinds of ligaments and are inherited through a specific identifiable gene. It is thought that rheumatoid arthritis has a genetic component, and we know that RA can cause back pain. The tendency to develop the crack in the back called spondylolysis, discussed earlier, may be inherited in some people. Finally, people with achondroplasia have a genetic condition that makes them prone to back problems and pain.

Even when all of these possibilities are taken into account, however, for most people with back pain, there probably is no defined gene to predict whether any one individual is more likely to have back pain than another.

Other Causes of Back Pain

As many people with back pain can attest, identifying the source of back pain is not always an easy or straightforward process. Pain in the back may be caused by a problem with the hips or pelvis, for example, and not by structures in the back at all. When a physician can't be sure what's causing the pain in the back (and therefore how to treat it), he or she has to do things differently in terms of the physical examination and diagnostic tests to identify the source of the pain.

A variety of other physical problems cause back pain, including abdominal aorta aneurysm, kidney stones, pelvic tumors, and problems with the pancreas, liver, or kidneys, and hip or sacroiliac arthritis.

Some people with hip arthritis hurt in their lower back. With referred pain from the hip, the sacroiliac joint, and elsewhere that

Back Pain at a Glance: Who Is at Risk for Back Pain?
- Anyone over the age of 30.
- Anyone with arthritis or osteoporosis.
- Women who have gone through menopause.
- Anyone who is not physically active.
- Any pregnant woman or new mother.
- Anyone with a health problem such as diabetes, hypertension, and cancer.
- Anyone who smokes.
- Anyone who has recently had surgery or is susceptible to infections.
- Anyone with a genetic tendency to develop back problems.

is felt in the back, the physician may perform a provocative physical examination (trying to provoke the pain during the exam) and may order bone scans or CT scans, plain x-rays, an MRI scan, and therapeutic injections such as a sacroiliac joint injection or a hip joint injection to determine the cause of the pain (see Chapter 8).

By the way, referred pain works in reverse, as well: There are spine conditions that can cause hip pain. Spine problems can cause leg weakness and hip pain from muscle imbalance. It can be difficult to find out why a person has hip pain and leg weakness. An MRI scan of the pelvis and the hip can be revealing, and physicians can also tell a lot by observing how a person walks (the gait pattern). The primary problem may be the back, but the back is causing weakness in the leg leading to hip pain. Treating this pain includes strengthening the back muscles, which leads to a normal gait and improvement in the hip.

In this chapter, we have described the variety of factors that determine who develops back pain, including age, lifestyle, general health, and genes. In Chapter 3, we take a closer look at some of the specific conditions that cause back pain.

Three
Things That Go Wrong in the Back

BACK PAIN COMES IN many varieties, from a dull ache to a sharp ache in the lower back to a pain down the leg or in your buttock. Back pain can show up as pain in places other than the back: in the knee, the hip, the buttock. Sometimes there is numbness rather than pain (or in addition to pain). Loss of function can be a more significant problem than pain. When nerves around the joints and discs are inflamed, weakness and numbness in the legs may develop. If the nerves are impinged, there may be problems with sexual function or loss of control or bladder function.

However, usually there is pain first. Finding out the cause of back pain can be challenging and sometimes involves several physicians and multiple diagnostic tests. By the time an experienced physician examines the patient, he or she often has a good idea of what's wrong before the test results. The physician will interpret the patient's symptoms using a step-by-step process, beginning with a thorough history followed by a physical examination and appropriate diagnostic studies. Although most back pain is related to normal aging, some people have a condition that requires immediate attention. The physician's role is to diagnose the cause of the pain and then recommend and arrange for treatment to try to relieve the symptoms and resolve the problem.

~hapter, we will look closely at the most common back
~~ ~ain, in the order of most common to least
~any of these conditions.) Cancer,
~~xt chapter.

age of conditions
nose but is usually
person stresses the
use of the pain could
its or tendons, or irri-
s understandable that
rce of the pain—a spe-
cific disc, ͟   wever, determining the
source may not be pᴜ͟

Soft tissue injuries are a comᴜ͟   e of back strain. Different types of soft tissue are attached to the spinal column, including muscles, ligaments, and joint capsules. There are ligaments between the spinous processes (the bones that stick out in the back of the spine). Strenuous activities can stretch those structures beyond their limits and can cause micro-tears in those structures. Alternatively, the structures simply are mechanically irritated and inflamed, which leads to back pain.

If the doctor tells the patient, "I believe that you have suffered lumbar sprain," and the patient asks, "What happened?" the doctor may say, "Well, it's possible that you tore a ligament or pulled a muscle, and that is the reason you hurt." Can the doctor diagnose this condition with imaging? Often the answer is no. Imaging capability for lumbar sprain is very poor, so we rule out possible causes. If the patient does not have a disc herniation, does not have a broken bone, and does not have any evidence of infection, and we know that the pain occurred because of activity, then the most likely diagnosis is lumbar sprain. In an extreme case, a small alteration may be seen in the muscle or the ligament on a magnetic resonance imaging (MRI) scan. However most of the time we can't see direct evidence of the cause even on an MRI scan. Therefore, after we rule out all the conditions that can be diagnosed, we say that the person has lumbar sprain. This description of the condition is as specific as the physician can be in explaining the cause of the symptoms.

Fortunately, back pain is usually a benign, self-limiting condition that resolves over time. In most cases, it should be treated with medications such as nonsteroidal anti-inflammatory medications. By reducing inflammation, these medications reduce the symptoms in the first ten days to two weeks. Other pain medications such as narcotics can also be useful in the early phase if the pain is severe. However, these medications can themselves cause problems, such as constipation, leading to more pain. Narcotics in particular can cause people to become lethargic and depressed, leading to less activity. Less activity is not desirable because people need to be as active as possible within the limits of their pain and need to gradually increase their activities over time (see Chapter 6).

It helps if patients keep in mind that lower back pain often takes several weeks to go away. If incapacitating pain disrupts your life, affecting your ability to stand, to sit, or to do normal activities, and if this is the first time you have had this pain, it can be very frightening. This is when people end up in the emergency room or seek treatment from their doctor. Be assured: in most cases, the pain will go away.

However, we acknowledge that back pain can be severe. You can't get out of bed, you can't work, you can't walk. A short period of rest—a couple of days—may be necessary, but then you need to return to your activities. Resuming activities is the appropriate approach; studies show that an early resumption of activities leads to less back pain and a shorter duration of back pain. In one study of army recruits who had back pain, one group of recruits was told to go to bed and stay in bed for a long time, and the other group was told to stay in bed for a short time and then get up, walk around, and get active. The group that returned to activity sooner got better more quickly and had an improved result than the people who remained on bed rest.

Gradually returning as quickly as possible to a normal level of activity is the best treatment for lumbar sprain. Inactivity is not good. We have learned the lesson from many conditions that inactivity is bad for us.

Herniated Disc (Slipped Disc or Vertebra)

When a person gets an MRI scan, a radiologist who examines the scan often will describe something called *disc bulge*, which in most instances is a normal part of the aging process and is not a sign of a problem or illness. In some instances, the jelly inside the disc squirts out through the outer layer and lodges or rests in the spinal canal and presses on the nerves, causing pain called *sciatica*.

The most common symptom of sciatica due to a herniated disc is pain that runs down the legs below the knees, following the distribution of a nerve root. Sciatica means pain due to irritation of one or more of the nerves that form the sciatic nerve, a major nerve that runs down the leg (see Figure 1). The pain can radiate all the way down to the foot. Generally, a herniated disc (also called a *ruptured*, or *slipped*, disc; see Figure 6) affects just one of those nerves, not more than one, and there are characteristic patterns of pain, numbness, weakness, or reflex changes that correspond to a particular nerve. People with disc herniation or disc problems often have a hard time sitting, bending forward, and driving (which involves both sitting and vibrating). These activities put a lot more pressure on the disc and can cause the disc fragment to bulge and press on the nerve.

With a herniated disc, the onset of symptoms can be sudden and associated with a physical event, or it can be gradual. As we noted in Chapter 2, that particular physical event is not necessarily the cause of the herniation, but it is the cause of the symptoms. Understandably, the patient associates the symptoms with that event. Often a twisting or bending activity leads to excruciating pain or numbness that runs down the person's leg in a particular pattern. But disc herniation is usually the result of degenerative disc disease, a process that has been ongoing for some time. In fact, many patients describe having vague back pain before the leg pain begins. Physicians hypothesize that the precursor pain is due to a piece of nucleus beginning to migrate through the anulus—that tirelike structure around the disc—and that the vague back pain is felt before the nucleus starts to pinch or irritate the nerve.

To diagnose a person who is describing the symptoms of a herniated disc, the physician performs a history and a physical examination. The physician asks the patient specific questions to identify the causes of the pain or what causes the pain to get worse:

- Does bending forward cause the pain?
- Does bending backward cause the pain?

When you bend forward, you load the disc, so many people with disc problems will be limited in bending forward. Bending forward will cause leg pain because the disc bulges more and presses on the nerve. Anything you do that stretches the nerve will cause an increase in pain. This is one of the classic signs of a disc herniation. One diagnostic test we use straightens the leg and then raises it straight up. This is called the *straight leg raise*. Many patients do the opposite of the straight leg test when they sleep at night. They will sleep on their side with their knees bent and their legs brought up in the fetal position. Or, while lying on their back, they will put several pillows under their knees, with their knees up, to relieve pressure and tension on the nerve by decreasing the stretch on it.

Another question the physician may ask is whether the pain increases when you cough, sneeze, or have a bowel movement. These activities increase the pressure on the nerve and cause pain.

Irritation to different nerves produces different patterns, some more obvious than others. The pattern of pain and numbness, weakness and reflexes often indicates which nerve root is affected. Compression of the S1 nerve root can cause pain that runs down the back of the leg to the bottom of the foot. There can be weakness in the gastrocnemius muscle, the muscle that allows us to rise up on our toes. Loss of sensation over the back of the leg and bottom of the foot can also be found by the physician. Irritation to this particular nerve can also cause a decrease in the Achilles reflex. Normally, when the physician hits the Achilles tendon, the foot goes down. However, when there is irritation of the S1 nerve, there can be a decrease in that reflex function.

By simply examining the patient and putting all this information together, the physician can determine that the S1 nerve root has likely been affected. A study such as an MRI scan can be used to confirm that the S1 nerve root is compressed, and the doctor can conclude confidently that the patient has a condition affecting the S1 nerve root, which causes all these problems.

Physicians then put everything together to make the diagnosis: the patient's history, the examination findings that identify which nerves are affected, and the MRI findings. Only when everything has been put together can the physician conclude, "Given all this information, I believe that this particular disc is herniated in this direction, affecting this nerve root and leading to this dysfunction."

If the MRI does not show the problem clearly, then additional tests, such as a myelogram and computerized tomography (CT) scan, EMG/nerve conduction study, and other tests may be needed. You cannot have an MRI if you have a pacemaker or certain implants. You may need a myelogram followed by a CT scan, which involves injecting dye through a lumbar puncture. (These procedures are described in detail in Chapter 5.)

Fortunately, most times a herniated disc will improve on its own, in about six to eight weeks. Nearly always, the majority of the leg pain will disappear and the back pain will improve. Pain occurs when the herniation first happens in part because of the inflammation associated with the disc rupture. The body reacts to this new piece of tissue being in the wrong spot. Over six to eight weeks, the size of the disc usually doesn't change, but the inflammation disappears, and when that occurs, the pain goes away and there is not enough mechanical pressure to cause pain. (Nerves can accommodate a certain amount of mechanical pressure without causing symptoms.)

Painful back spasms can also occur with disc herniation. The spasm means the body is trying to splint the disc with muscles or position the vertebrae in a way that will relieve pressure on the nerves. Muscle relaxants are often useful in relieving back spasms. If we are certain about which disc is herniated, and if the symptoms are not improving, we may consider a surgical procedure called a *discectomy* to relieve the pain.

Spinal Stenosis

Spinal stenosis is a condition in which the tunnel where the nerves travel becomes narrowed. It is usually due to arthritis and typically begins to affect people in their fifties, increasing in incidence as people age. It is more likely to happen in people born with a smaller channel for the nerves, who then develop arthritis or a bulging of the disc that takes up more space where the nerves travel. But it can happen to anyone, regardless of how much space they are born with.

The typical symptoms of spinal stenosis are a feeling of pain, numbness, and weakness in the legs when standing or walking. Most people feel fine when they sit—their symptoms go away. They feel worse the longer they stand or the farther they walk, and they have the desire to sit down or lean forward to feel better and walk longer. They may feel comfortable and can stand and walk longer in a grocery store leaning over a shopping cart, for example. Spinal stenosis is a progressive disorder and gradually gets worse over time.

Put another way, we say that spinal stenosis causes *neurogenic claudication* (*neurogenic* = the nervous system; *claudication* = limping) because of nerve impingement. You may have no significant discomfort when you are seated, but when you stand or walk, you may experience fatigue, numbness, or pain radiating down the legs. The explanation for this pattern is that the spinal canal—the tunnel where the nerves run—narrows in the standing position and expands when you are seated or bent forward, so people are relieving the pressure on their nerves and relieving their symptoms by sitting or leaning forward.

There are well-recognized ways to accommodate to this condition: a cane or walker to lean forward on; sitting down frequently, if you are at a party, for example; and leaning on a shopping cart, which allows you to walk longer before you have to stop and sit down. The surgical treatment for neurogenic claudication is a *lumbar laminectomy*—the "unroofing of the nerves," which is described in Chapter 9.

Vascular Claudation

Vascular claudication produces symptoms that are almost identical to the symptoms of neurogenic claudication. This condition is not a compression of the nerves but rather a narrowing of blood vessels that travel to legs. Unlike neurogenic claudication, people with vascular claudication have to stop walking (they do not have to sit down) for the leg weakness and pain to go away. As long as you are not using your muscles, the muscles will recover. Symptoms occur because not enough blood reaches the muscles when the muscles are used for walking. Also the symptoms for vascular claudication tend to progress from the feet to the back. In neurogenic claudication, the symptoms start in the back and progress down the leg. So the direction of the symptoms is different.

One test to distinguish between the two conditions is the bicycle test. A person riding a bicycle is essentially in a seated position. Commonly a person with neurogenic claudication can function quite well in the seated position and riding the bike, whereas the person with vascular claudication will get muscle ischemia due to blood supply insufficiency and will not be able to keep bicycling. Many people with neurogenic claudication can bicycle for miles but, sadly, they aren't able to walk 100 feet.

To treat neurogenic claudication nonsurgically, we recommend anti-inflammatory medications such as nonsteroidal anti-inflammatory drugs as well as back exercises, emphasizing flexion exercises and abdominal muscle strengthening exercises. Epidural injections (see Chapter 6) may provide relief in the early stages of the condition. The success rate in surgery is very high, and the outcome is good with low complications.

Degenerative Spondylolisthesis

In the condition called *degenerative spondylolisthesis*, the arthritic process leads to a forward slippage of one vertebra on the other (see Figure 6). It can occur in association with spinal stenosis and may require additional surgery beyond a laminectomy.

The surgical procedure known as laminectomy inherently takes some of the support away from the spine, and if there is already some slippage of one vertebra onto another, performing a laminectomy often makes the condition worse by taking away some of the structural support of the spine. This leads to spinal instability and continued or worsening pain. Since a simple laminectomy for a person with degenerative spondylolisthesis may worsen the condition, particularly slippage leading to sciatica and mechanical back pain, a patient with degenerative spondylolisthesis often requires a fusion at the time of the laminectomy to hold the vertebrae together. The danger of not fusing is that there will be further slippage of one vertebra on the other, back pain, a return of the nerve pain, and the need for further surgery. (See Chapter 9.)

Spondylolysis

As noted in Chapter 2, spondylolysis is a crack or fracture in the pars interarticularis, the thin bridge of bone joining the lamina and inferior articular facet to the pedicle and superior facet. This condition can occur early in life, while a person is still growing, and often is not the result of trauma. If it newly develops in an adult, it is generally caused by trauma. Whether spondylolysis is acquired early or later in life from trauma, it occurs most often at the L5 vertebra. This leads to forward slippage of the L5 vertebra with respect to the sacrum. The crack, then, leads to spondylolisthesis, which is the slipping forward of one vertebra on another. Spondylolysis is illustrated in Figure 6.

Spondylolysis is a common condition: Between 8 and 12 percent of the population have it, although many people don't know they have it and have never had any significant back pain related to it. People such as gymnasts who hyperextend put a lot of stress on their backs and are more likely to develop spondylolysis or develop symptoms from this condition. When spondylolysis causes symptoms, the symptoms include back pain that can be associated with leg pain because of irritation of the nerves that run by the crack. The forward slippage allowed by the crack may result in loss of normal orientation of one vertebra to another, malalignment of the spine, nerve irritation due to nerve pressure, and back pain. One symptom that helps to identify a stress fracture is pain that worsens from bending back and standing.

Probably what most people think about stress fractures is that the bone can't take the repeated stress. Bones can remodel, strengthen, and tolerate stress without injury, but bones can't withstand a certain amount of increased load or stress unless the bone becomes stronger, when it can tolerate the load and not develop an injury from it. But when you rapidly increases the load on a bone, then the bone can't adapt to it and you may develop a stress fracture, which can happen in any bone in the body. Conceivably, if you went from no typing to typing 800 pages a day, you could get stress fractures in the fingers. Or, if a runner went from running twenty miles a week to sixty miles a week, stress fractures in the feet or shins could develop.

Many professional baseball players have suffered stress fractures—of the shinbone, for example—and many gymnasts have had a stress fracture at one time or another, as well. Gymnasts, ballet dancers, football linemen—people who hyperextend their back—can have a stress fracture. When gymnasts come down from a height and they need to land and maintain a perfect posture, the sheer force applies directly to the pars, which can break. They flip and hyperextend their backs or they do a reverse handstand and flip back on the balance beam, while holding onto the balance beam. Floor exercises can also strain the spinal column. Most people, of course, are not loading their spines to that degree.

Stress fractures are *fractures*—they are broken bones—but they are broken bones that occur not from a single event but rather from repetitive overloading of a bone. The bone does not repair itself and get stronger. (When we allow the bone to repair itself, it can tolerate the stress without injury when it encounters that load repeatedly.) The bone is just as broken as if you'd fallen off the curb and broken an ankle. However, what causes the break are many little injuries from which it can never recover as opposed to a single load that overwhelms it (such as falling off a curb). Stress fractures tend to be hairline fractures and often are not displaced (the bone does not shift its position), at least not initially.

Back pain from stress fractures is more prevalent in younger people who have had back pain off and on since adolescence. Symptoms come from the crack in the bone. Leg pain is more common for people in their forties or fifties who are starting to develop arthritis and disc degeneration; the crack accelerates the disc degeneration because the disc has to absorb the entire load of the spine. Furthermore, the body's attempts to heal the crack produce scar tissue in the foramen, and then the disc bulges and narrows the space even more so that stenosis pinches the nerves.

Plain x-rays and CT, MRI, and bone scans are useful in diagnosing spondylolysis. A hairline fracture often is not visible on plain x-rays, but a CT scan and bone scan can detect it. A bone scan identifies areas where bone cells are trying to repair fractures and highlights a specific area of the bone. CT scans are useful for looking at bones in different planes to pinpoint a hairline fracture. MRI scans can be useful in visualizing nerve compression and seeing edema in soft tissues and bone. (See Chapter 5 for a description of these tests.)

The initial treatment is to cut down on the physical training and let the back heal. Sometimes a back brace is used to provide support and to help the back rest. Other treatments include anti-inflammatory medications and back and abdominal strengthening exercises, including psoas stretching exercises. Injections of steroids and local anesthetic into the foramen (called *foramenal injections*) can be used to bathe the affected nerve. Steroids are used to try to reduce the inflammation, and anesthetic temporarily relieves pain (see Chapter 6).

Spondylosis

Spondylosis is a degenerative disease of the spinal column that leads to immobility and stiffness. Simply put, it is degenerative arthritis—the same arthritis that can occur in any joint in the body.

Scoliosis

Scoliosis is a twisting of the spine in multiple planes that leads to an abnormal curvature of the spinal column. Although there may be a familial tendency to scoliosis, even after years of research we still don't know what causes scoliosis. We cannot describe the genetic component and whether other components are more important than genetics in developing scoliosis.

Scoliosis screening for preadolescents (in the 12-year-old range) started in school systems over thirty years ago and has led to a significant reduction in the number of people requiring surgery. If scoliosis is suspected, then the child or adolescent is referred to a physician for evaluation and treatment.

In a person with scoliosis, the vertebral bodies are turned with respect to each other, so the spine twists like a corkscrew. People who have curves in their backs may notice that their shoulders and hips are uneven. They lose their waistline. One part of their rib cage will be more prominent than the other, and their pants length or hemline is uneven. Pain is relatively rare for people with scoliosis.

Back Pain at a Glance: What Do People Notice When They Are Getting Scoliosis or When Scoliosis Is Getting Worse?

- They notice an asymmetry—a shifting of their body—of their shoulders over their pelvis. They may notice one leg is shorter than the other. Their pants leg or hemline may be significantly shorter on one side than on the other.
- When they have progression, which is an increase in the size or shape of the curve, patients often notice that they have to change their hemline or change their pants length frequently.
- They may notice that they have a change in or even lost their waist.
- Adults will have difficulty standing up straight. They may be told to stand up straight, to straighten their shoulders out, or to straighten their hips out, and they will not be able to do it.
- Scoliosis can be associated with kyphosis—a forward bending of the spine. People with kyphosis often have to bend their knees to look straight ahead. If their knees are straight and locked and their hips are straight, they will be looking at the ground.
- People who have adult scoliosis may notice back fatigue, generally on one side of their spine and not the other. For many people, arthritis starts on the concave side of the curve, and then as arthritis develops, it spreads to the convex side of the curve.
- People notice that their pain is relieved if they lie down, if they get traction, or if they stretch their spine out by lifting their trunk with their arms when sitting.
- Adults with pain notice that the pain gets worse over the course of the day and depending on how long they stand and that it will be relieved by lying down or sitting down.

For adolescent girls, scoliosis may affect their body image, especially at such a sensitive time in their development. So treatment often addresses both self-image and medical needs. Although cosmetic considerations do not drive surgeons to recommend an operation, they may be the main reason a patient asks a doctor to perform an operation. Physical attractiveness is an important benchmark for a patient's satisfaction or lack of satisfaction with an operation.

There are three main types of scoliosis:

1. *Juvenile scoliosis* is relatively rare (and not relevant to this book) and involves a scoliosis that develops in young children. It tends to be severe and often is not responsive to bracing.

2. *Idiopathic scoliosis* is associated with growth and is the most common type of scoliosis (*idiopathic* means "no known cause"). It occurs more often in girls than in boys during the adolescent growth spurt. Scoliosis is not caused by poor posture, lack of calcium, or playing sports. Nor will good posture, plenty of calcium, or not playing sports change the course of scoliosis.

Idiopathic scoliosis does not usually cause pain. Scoliosis in a growing child has the capacity to get worse very quickly, and someone who is still growing is at risk for increasing deformity.

Bracing during the critical growth period can minimize the progress of scoliosis, and a child who otherwise would require surgery may be able to avoid an operation if the condition is caught and braced early. This is why school screening and early recognition of scoliosis is critical.

Typically, braces are given to children and adolescents who are at risk for progression. Then the patient is followed up on a regular schedule determined by the size and type of the curve and its response to treatment. There are ways of using x-rays of the hand and pelvis to see growth pattern and skeletal maturity. X-rays are useful in determining whether or how often to screen someone, whether they need bracing, and when to stop the bracing.

When a child or adolescent is diagnosed with scoliosis, physicians collect a family history of the condition as part of the medical history: Do aunts or uncles, parents or grandparents have scoliosis? The physician will especially examine siblings—sisters in particular—because females are more likely than males to have scoliosis. Siblings who are diagnosed with the disease may also be treated with bracing.

Treating scoliosis involves measuring the spinal curve in degrees. A very minor curve is not necessarily scoliosis. A curve must be greater than 10 degrees before it is considered scoliosis. In general, if you have a curve measured between 10 and 20 degrees, then we probably do not need to do anything about it other than follow the patient closely to see whether the curve progresses. If you have a curve between 20 and 30 degrees, a doctor may recommend bracing. Someone with a curve greater than 30 degrees needs to be followed closely and may need to wear a brace for a short period. If there is progression, then surgery may be necessary. If the curve is 75 degrees or greater, lung function can be affected and surgery may be necessary.

The braces for treating scoliosis partially straighten out the curve and need to be worn for long periods—most of the day and night—to be effective. The brace will push the ribs and the spine into a more neutral position as growth occurs, which allows for normal growth or at least prevents the curve from progressing. Braces are not uncomfortable, but they are stiff and limiting. Self-image is a significant problem because braces are bulky and make the wearer appear heavier than he or she is. Some people fail to wear their braces as prescribed (they are noncompliant), both because of cosmesis (appearance) and because of discomfort.

It is critical to see a recognized scoliosis specialist for medical treatment. Scoliosis experts tend to be pediatric orthopedic surgeons with an interest in spine surgery and orthopedic spine surgeons, even though surgery is less common now because of improved early screening and a better understanding of treating scoliosis nonoperatively. Patients must see the specialist frequently, particularly if they are braced, to determine whether the brace is effective and whether the curve is progressing. Deciding about intervening surgically is a complex process; therefore, having a physician with experience in treating scoliosis is essential.

3. *Adult scoliosis* develops after the person's skeleton is fully mature. Adults may develop a new curve, or an existing curve may get worse as arthritic processes continue. That is, they either develop

scoliosis as a new condition due to the arthritis and the wear and tear on the back or as an increase in symptoms of scoliosis left over from childhood. As older people with scoliosis develop severe arthritic changes in their spinal column and in their hips, an existing scoliosis can progress because of the arthritis, and scoliosis can accelerate the arthritis and degeneration in other parts of their spinal column as well.

Bracing does not work to correct the curve in adults because adults are not growing. Nonoperative measures are used to treat adults with symptoms from scoliosis because of pain and nerve symptoms. If the symptoms don't improve or if the curve increases, you must consider surgery. The surgical procedure is designed to straighten out the curve as best as possible, remove the pressure on the nerves (which is an important component of the pain), and then stabilize the curve in a functionally acceptable position.

Fusions with instrumentation that partially correct the scoliotic curve are a common form of surgical treatment (see Chapter 9), with the addition of osteotomies, in which parts of the bone are removed and wedges are created in the bone to straighten out the spine. This surgery is neither easy to perform nor easy to undergo. Therefore, a person in need of this procedure must find a surgeon who performs it frequently. Many complex spine surgeries involving kyphosis or scoliosis are complicated and lengthy procedures. It can take up to a full year to recover and can involve a hospital stay of up to several weeks with a rehabilitation stay afterward. On the plus side, most people will notice immediately that they are standing up straighter, that the pains in their legs are gone, and that they have a significant improvement in their overall balance and an improvement in the shape of their body.

To reiterate: It can take up to a year to recover from the complex spine surgery needed to address spinal curvature in an adult.

Weakened Bones from Steroid Treatment

Steroids are a blessing for many people with medical conditions whose symptoms respond to steroids and sometimes little else. But steroids are also a problem because high doses break down bone. Bone loss is not uncommon in people after chronic steroid use,

Back Pain at a Glance: When Should Children, Adolescents, and Adults Consider Surgery for Scoliosis?

The criteria for deciding to operate are different for each of the three types of scoliosis. We cannot apply the reasoning and rationales used to make decisions for one type to another type.

- Juvenile (childhood) scoliosis is a complex disease that requires an expert's guidance, and those experts are pediatric orthopedic surgeons who specialize in scoliosis. Since juveniles progress rapidly and often have an associated congenital issue that can worsen with growth, juveniles with smaller magnitudes of curves tend to be operated on more frequently than people with other types of scoliosis.
- In adolescence, the issues are:
  1. How large is the curve?
  2. How much growth remains?
  3. What type of curve is it, and is it amenable to a brace?
  4. How does it respond to treatment? Does it stay the same or get better with the brace?

  If the curve responds to bracing and the child is nearly finished growing, these tend to be reasons not to operate. If the curve worsens, then surgery may be necessary.
- In adults, bracing is not an effective form of treatment for the curve. Treatment tends to focus on improving symptoms such as nerve pain and back pain from arthritis. These symptoms are treated with physical therapy, pain medications, anti-arthritic medications, and in some instances, selective blocks such as epidurals and nerve root blocks with cortisone. Two basic reasons for surgery in adults are:
  1. Symptoms affecting quality of life.
  2. Curve magnitude and progression, affecting quality of life and predicting poor quality of life in the future if not treated.

  If the curve affects the person's ability to stand or walk for any distance, if it is causing pain that cannot be controlled by nonoperative means, or if it is rapidly increasing its size (curve progression), these are reasons for surgery. Most surgeons will not operate on patients for strictly cosmetic reasons. However, many *patients* find the surgery appealing for the cosmetic improvement and find cosmesis rather than alleviation of the symptoms to be a reason for having it done or a reason for satisfaction with the results.

such as people who've had heart transplant or a kidney transplant surgery who take high doses of steroids to suppress their immune system so their new organ will not be rejected. Steroids are also commonly used to suppress inflammation in the joints and other parts of the body in people with rheumatoid arthritis. A person with bronchial asthma or chronic pulmonary disease often needs steroids to suppress allergic reaction so they can breathe properly. All these diseases may require high doses of steroids to treat the underlying condition, but long-term use of steroids leads to osteoporosis and eventually, when the bones are under stress and under load, they break or fracture. People with osteoporosis from steroid use can develop *compression fractures* of their spinal column (see Chapter 2).

Unfortunately, it is not easy for some people to stop taking steroids because they are so dependent on the medication for other health reasons, and the longer they take steroids, the more their bones break down. Steroid-induced osteoporosis tends to be pronounced with a higher risk of fractures, and treatment is extremely difficult. Going off high-dose steroids reverses some of the effects of the medication but not necessarily the osteoporosis that it created.

Infection

Infection is an uncommon cause of pain in the back. Infection can occur after spine surgery or other spine procedures such as a discogram or biopsy. Infection can also start somewhere else. People who have recently had a tooth infection (a tooth abscess), a urinary tract infection, or some sort of sepsis can develop an infection that lodges in the spine.

The characteristic symptoms of back infections are *nonmechanical* back pain; that is, back pain that occurs no matter what position the person is in and won't go away with rest. The pain also tends to be *unrelenting* and *progressive*. People have problems with pain at night and problems sleeping. *Fever, chills, and night sweats* can be signs of infection in the back. An infection in the back may be misdiagnosed as a sprain, or, if there is fever, it may be misdiagnosed as pneumonia, urinary tract infection, or some other infection.

Infections in the spine are difficult to diagnose because they produce few if any specific signs or symptoms that point to an infection, except for steadily increasing, unrelenting pain. (*Symptoms* are problems noticed and reported by the patient; *signs* are findings noted by the physician when examining the patient.) The average delay in diagnosis is long: A person may have several weeks up to several months of back pain without a correct diagnosis of infection. This is an unsafe situation because, as we will see, one key to treating back infection is an early diagnosis.

Infections tend to occur in the disc from different bacteria that invade the disc and erode the vertebral bodies next to the disc. This erosion can lead to the collapse of the vertebral bodies from the weakening of the bones involved in the infection. The concern with a back infection is nerve damage and paralysis from developing a large abscess or pocket of pus that causes pressure and other damage to the spinal nerves and the spinal cord. That situation, in combination with any bone collapsing, can cause permanent paralysis. Neurological injuries can develop very suddenly and rapidly due to vascular infarcts of the nerves; this means that the blood supply to the nerves dies, so the paralysis is not reversible. This process is like having a heart attack of the spinal cord: The nerves die because blood does not supply them.

When the infection is diagnosed early, the treatment involves identifying the organism, protecting or immobilizing the back with a brace if possible, and giving antibiotics—usually IV antibiotics—usually for six weeks to three months until the infection is resolved. When the infection is advanced and there is either pressure on the nerves, bone destruction and collapse, or failure of treatment with antibiotics, then surgery is necessary to remove the infected tissue and stabilize the infected joint through a fusion. This surgery is typically done from the front; the disc is removed, the infected material is removed, and a bone graft is placed in the front and stabilized (either with an external brace or plates, screws, and rods). The surgery is followed by antibiotics for six weeks to three months or longer.

Infections in the spine generally start in the disc space and then spread to the bone (bone infection is called *osteomyelitis*). Disc infections may be isolated, but most commonly, by the time they are diagnosed, the adjacent bone is involved (osteomyelitis). Antibiotics and bracing have proved to be effective in treating back infections in the early stages, before there is much bone erosion.

The role of the brace is to reduce pain, hold the back in position, and keep it from collapsing. There are different types of braces, including braces that look like a clamshell made of plastic and others that have pads on the chest and pubis and straps around the back to try to hold the spine still. Bracing prevents the bone from collapsing further and reduces the pain from motion. In instances in which the bones have collapsed, bracing alone does not restore a normal shape to the spine, and surgery is often needed to restore and maintain the spine. Surgery is performed in addition to antibiotics.

Tuberculosis is a different kind of an infection that involves the vertebral bodies first; the disc spaces are preserved. The vertebral bodies are a good environment for infection because they provide a rich source of nutrients. Tuberculosis infection is more readily treated with antibiotics and bracing than some other infections.

Back Pain at a Glance: What Should People Think about If They Have Any Kind of Infection Followed by Back Pain?
Because the key to treating back infections successfully is early diagnosis, here are some things for people to think about:

- If you have had an infection of any sort—a sinus infection, for example, or a urinary tract infection, pneumonia, or abscess followed by tooth extraction—and then you develop back pain seemingly for no reason, and the back pain continues for more than a few weeks without letting up, you may have an infection in your back, and you should see a doctor as soon as possible.

- If you have had a urinary tract manipulation—such as a urethral dilation procedure (where the physician stretches the urethra with an instrument), a bladder operation, or a cystoscopic procedure—you may develop an infection such as cystitis. If you had this procedure within a several-month window before the acute onset of low back pain, you may have an infection in the back and you should see a doctor as soon as possible.

- If you have an infection in another location—an abscess that has been drained, pneumonia that has been treated, or an infected pimple that was popped—and then you develop back pain seemingly for no reason, and the back pain continues for more than several weeks without letting up, you may have an infection in your back, and you should see a doctor as soon as possible.

Many people get back infections from blood-borne channels and are very sick. They may have a urinary tract infection (UTI), and their back infection is misdiagnosed as UTI alone; the UTI may subside, but the back pain continues. Or they may have renal failure, or a compromised immune system (from chemotherapy for cancer treatment, for example, or from AIDS), and the infection is quite serious and can threaten their neurological function (for example, if the infection is in the lumbar region, it may affect their bowel or bladder control). Such infections can be serious and potentially life threatening.

A person can get an infection from a discogram or other diagnostic studies in which a needle is inserted into the disc to determine pain (see Chapter 5). Infection is rare, but if it happens, it can be painful and potentially severe.

Many patients with discitis need to be admitted to the hospital to control their pain because pain control requires IV narcotics. These patients are placed in braces, which are also helpful in alleviating their pain. Physicians must establish the diagnosis, and to find out which particular bacteria or other agents caused the infection, physicians rely on biopsies of the disc space. They usually use CT-guided approaches in radiology to place the needle into the disc space to aspirate fluid and do a culture. Based on the culture results, the patient will be started on appropriate antibiotics. If the results are inconclusive, then the physician will do blood cultures: Blood from the patient is grown in a growth medium, and if the growth is positive, it generally indicates the type of bacteria, which the physician can treat. A person with a back infection needs to be treated for six to eight weeks at least, if not longer. Because the antibiotics must be administered by IV, a long-term IV-access line is placed in the patient's body, so that the patient can receive antibiotics at home.

We follow a number of markers in the blood to diagnose infection as well as follow the patient's response to treatment. The common markers are erythrocyte sedimentation rate and C-reactive protein. These are nonspecific markers of inflammation in the body and are usually elevated in patients with discitis. After the patient has been on antibiotics, those numbers gradually come down. We periodically check them to make sure that the patient is responding to the treatment. How much pain the patient has, and whether the patient is feeling better, is another indication of response to the therapy. If the pain is improving, that's a significant indication of a response to therapy.

In addition to at least six to eight weeks of antibiotic treatment, the patient wears a brace, which is helpful in alleviating the pain. Many patients develop a fusion on their own in the disc space as a result of infection, and when the fusion occurs, usually the pain is gone. (A fusion is the growing together of two vertebrae.) The infection can lead to the destruction of the vertebral bodies above, and in this situation, the patient may develop angulation of the spinal column, or kyphosis, and may need a major reconstructive procedure, often from both the front and the back.

Epidural abscesses are infections of the space in the spinal canal that the spinal cord and nerves usually occupy. These abscesses can happen spontaneously or can happen in association with another infection. They may occur when discitis or osteomyelitis spreads to the spinal canal. They are more likely to develop in people with a history of IV drug abuse, in people whose immune systems are compromised either from disease such as HIV or from chemotherapy, and in people with kidney failure. These conditions can set up an ideal environment for infection. Postoperative spine surgery patients are at high risk as well. If the patient has many ongoing infections, and the patient is not strong, epidural abscesses are more likely. A pharynx infection—a strep or staph infection in the head and neck—sometimes spreads to the cervical area. Sometimes pharyngeal infections after head or neck surgery from the tonsils or an abscess behind the throat are severe and can extend out to the spinal canal, which is located right behind the throat.

An epidural abscess can spread quickly like a wildfire up and down the spine, traveling through the blood vessels that line the spinal canal. Like appendicitis, it is a serious, true emergency. A surgeon will operate to try to eradicate the infection as rapidly as possible for several reasons: (1) it can press on the nerves, causing compression and malfunctioning of the nerves; (2) it can continue to spread rapidly; and (3) because of the possibility of infarct—the death of the nerves from a lack of blood supply (the blood supply is cut off by the inflammation at the site of the infection and by the mechanical pressure of the infection). For these reasons, despite the surgeon's best efforts to remove the infection as quickly as possible, if the blood vessels are already inflamed and the blood supply to the spinal cord is already cut off, there may be irreversible or permanent neurological deficits and paralysis.

Back Pain at a Glance: What Are the Most Common Conditions That Cause Back Pain?
- Lumbar sprain
- Spondylolysis
- Herniated disc (slipped disc)
- Spinal stenosis
- Degenerative spondylolisthesis
- Spondylosis
- Scoliosis
- Infection
- Traumatic fracture
- Tumor

Traumatic Fractures

Traumatic fractures are more likely to occur in working age or young adults—in people who are in the most productive times of their lives. Fractures stemming from falls or car accidents are potentially devastating and life altering. Fractures tend to occur right at the transition area from the rigid thoracic spine to the mobile lumbar spine because the body's biomechanics put a lot of stress on that area. This is where the spinal cord is about to end, so when there is a fracture in that area, an injury to nerves can occur.

Dislocations of the joints can also occur as part of a traumatic injury. In some traumatic incidents, damage is limited to a broken bone, while in others there is also either partial or complete injury of the spinal cord because broken bones can press on the nerves of the spinal cord and sometimes sever them. If this happens, either weakness in the lower extremities or complete paralysis can occur.

Treatment of spine fractures can range from bracing to complex surgery. Treatment depends on the type of fracture, whether there is a nerve injury associated with the fracture, and the type and cause of the nerve injury.

Surgery requires removing broken bones, reestablishing the normal contour of the spine, and supporting the bones with additional bones or metallic devices such as screws and rods. Usually, the area will fuse, and the spine will take from about three to six months to as long as a year to heal. Eventually, it will support the patient's weight and protect the spinal cord, and the patient's pain will diminish.

Four

Spinal Tumors and Metastatic Cancer

IN THE SIMPLEST OF terms, cancer is uncontrolled division of a cell. Under normal circumstances, we have cells in our body that divide on a regular basis. We have checks and balances in place that control that growth; however, we don't let cells grow too fast. Occasionally, the cells get out of control, and then our immune system selectively detects those cells and kills them. All of us actually have cancer forming in our body many times a day. As you read this page, your gut is creating cancer, your lungs are creating cancer, and your skin is dividing and forming cancer. As long as you have a strong immune system and the checks and balances are operational, the cancer cells will not last. Your body will selectively find and kill them.

The problem comes in when the body's checks and balances are not working well. Either the immune system or the internal mechanisms that control the growth of a given cell are not working well. It is possible that because of your genetic predisposition your mechanisms to control cell growth were already prone not to work ideally, and then something else happens—an injury to the cell from a virus, let's say—and eventually the cells get out of control. For that to happen, there must be more than one failure in controlling the cell—it cannot be just a single failure, which is rare. For a tumor to form and to grow, the cells must have multiple mechanisms that are not working well. Physicians can prescribe drugs to attack the specific out-of-control pathways.

One difficulty about cancer is you never really know whether you have been cured, and even if you are cured, the disease and its treatment have such a profound effect on your life. Growing evidence suggests that cancer eventually will become a chronic disease, such as high blood pressure or diabetes. You will be able to take a handful of medications (not one, but five or six) to affect specific pathways in a given cell to control disease. An example of this approach is the treatment for AIDS. Five or six categories of medications attack the virus that causes AIDS in multiple sites; eventually, these medications will be strong enough to kill the virus. The same is likely to happen in cancer treatment.

Cancer is serious, and there are tragic stories of young people dying from primary spinal cord tumors. Many patients do well; their tumor is completely removed, and they return to running marathons. Sometimes the tumor is large, and the expectation after surgery is that the patient might no longer be able to walk or have bowel or bladder control or sexual function. But such predictions do not always come true, and the patient can have normal function after surgery. Sometimes multiple operations are needed to remove a tumor that comes back repeatedly after surgery. And sometimes a cancer diagnosis is missed. You may have tingling in your hands and be told you have carpal tunnel syndrome when you actually have a spinal tumor.

Sometimes surgery is the only way to know that a patient has a malignant tumor. We have seen patients who were diagnosed with malignant tumors; when we operated, the tumors turned out not to be malignant. The patient will have had imaging studies, such as an MRI, or a CT scan, but only surgery that provides direct access to the tissue gives us a definitive diagnosis. We have operated on patients who have had radiation therapy to relieve pain from an "inoperable" tumor, and we were convinced from x-rays and scans that the tumor was malignant, and then, in rare and exceptional circumstances, we find that the tumor is benign and could be resected completely. (*Resect* means to remove surgically.)

We cannot always determine from x-ray and scans that the patient can or cannot benefit from surgery. This is an essential concept: Diagnosis cannot be made from imaging tests alone to conclude that a patient cannot benefit from surgery. A physician must be 100 percent sure that a patient cannot benefit from surgery. (As we will discuss, there *are* circumstances in which surgery is not an option, such as when the patient is not strong enough.)

Tumors can affect the bony components of the spinal column (the vertebral bodies, facet joints, spinal processes, lamina), or they can originate from within the spinal canal, from the neural structures or the tissues that cover them. And finally, they can arise from the structures near the spinal column and secondarily involve the spine. A good example would be a lung cancer that extended into the chest wall and then traveled into the spine. In this case, the spine happens to be the structure adjacent to the original site of the cancer.

When we consider tumors that originate in the spinal column, we consider them in two different categories. One category is primary tumors, which we will briefly discuss here. One of the most common tumors in young people is *osteoid-osteoma*, a benign tumor located inside a bone. This type of tumor can cause significant pain at night, but the pain responds to aspirin or ibuprofen. Findings on a CT scan, MRI, and bone scan usually are classic for this particular kind of tumor. One way to treat this type of tumor is with percutaneous ablation. The tumor has a core, and the surgeon uses a hot instrument to "fry" that area (this is called *percutaneous radiofrequency ablation*). Sometimes the tumor comes back and must be treated again.

As a rule, we do not do CT-guided biopsies of spinal cord tumors (tumors inside the covering of the spinal cord); a biopsy is done only after the tumor is exposed during surgery and before it is removed. A biopsy is, however, done in almost every case when the tumor is located outside the spinal cord (within the spinal column) or when the tumor has arisen in the tissue outside the spinal column.

Tumors that make up the largest category are the metastatic tumors that come to the spinal column from somewhere else. Metastatic disease affects older people more often than younger people, while primary spine tumors affect young people more often than older people.

Metastatic Cancer

Advances in medical care are making it possible for people to survive much longer after developing cancer. One consequence of lengthened survival is that people are living long enough to develop metastatic disease. In women, breast cancer is the most common source of tumor metastases to the spine. In men, the most common sources are lung cancer and prostate cancer. All cancers, including colon and thyroid cancer, can go to the spinal column and cause metastases, but the top three are breast cancer, lung cancer, and prostate cancer.

Bones are a common location for metastatic disease, and the spine is one of the more common places to get it. When these tumors go to the spinal column, they cause a number of problems.

1. There is pain from the tumor growing within the bone and stretching the membrane that covers the bone, which is sensitive to pain. Patients are in severe, relentless, local, nagging pain that is worse at night and that wakes them from their sleep, and they cannot find a comfortable sleeping position. People tend to see the doctor because of the pain.

2. The tumors destroy the vertebral bodies and therefore the vertebra fractures or collapses, which also creates pain. The pain in this situation is a bit different, in that, like any broken bone, it is related to the position of the patient. If you are trying to get up and walk, the pain worsens. Then when you lie down, the pain recedes. Pain related to the tumor growing and stretching the membrane responds to treatment modalities, such as steroids; radiation therapy, if the tumor happens to be sensitive to that treatment; or chemotherapy, if the tumor is likely to respond to that. But the mechanical pain—the pain that is related to broken bones in the spinal column—is resistant to these types of therapies. Patients with this type of pain most commonly need to be treated surgically; that area needs to be repaired, the tumor needs to be removed, and the spine needs to be stabilized. Here, a surgical approach effectively helps to control the patient's pain.

3. A growing tumor can put pressure on the nerves because either the tumor takes up space within the spinal canal or it causes a breakage of the bone, so that the bones go into the space where the spinal cord nerves are located. The pressure in turn may lead to weakness in both legs, impairment of bowel or bladder function, and impaired sexual function. This is a secondary problem called *epidural spinal cord compression* from the tumor. It is an urgent situation because if it is not treated quickly and effectively the patients progress—and they sometimes progress very rapidly—to complete loss of function in the legs and loss of bowel and bladder control.

Thus, treatment depends on what is causing the pressure on the spinal cord. If it is a tumor growing and the tumor happens to be sensitive to a specific treatment, we can treat it with radiation or chemotherapy, but if the problem is primarily mechanical or the tumor is not responsive to other treatment modalities, then it needs to be surgically treated. The operation gets rid of the tumor to take pressure off the nerves, to reconstruct the area of the spine, and then to stabilize things. We also commonly use steroids in conjunction with other therapies because steroids are effective in relieving the swelling that occurs from pressure on the nerves; steroids can protect the spinal cord function for a short time and effectively relieve pain in this situation.

Some tumors, such as metastases from renal cell cancer (a tumor that originates in the kidney), are highly vascular (they have a rich blood supply). These tumors commonly require surgery because they do not respond as well to other treatments. To minimize the risk of blood loss, a day or two before surgery, we perform a procedure called *embolization*. In an embolization, the blood vessels are injected, and the vessels that feed the tumor are seen and are, using particles, individually blocked off by the radiologist before the surgical intervention.

Most surgeries for metastatic disease in the spine are performed for palliative purposes—to relieve the patient's pain and to protect the patient's neurological function. When we operate on a patient with metastatic disease, we are addressing quality-of-life issues. Rarely do we perform an operation in the spinal column for metastatic disease with the intent of prolonging the patient's life because life expectancy is mostly determined by the extent of the disease and how well it can be treated. Patients may think, "Well, since everything has been taken care of, I am now going to live a normal life." They do not always grasp that the operation has a specific purpose, which is to offer a patient palliation for pain control and neurological preservation. This goal is entirely different in patients with primary spinal tumors (discussed in the next section).

Most metastatic disease involves anterior vertebral bodies (the front of the spine), but it can grow within the posterior elements of the spine. Spinal surgery for metastatic disease usually involves removing the tumor and then replacing the removed bone with implants or bone screws and rods to hold the spine still and secure. It can involve surgeries from the front of the spine, through the chest or through the abdomen, through the back or midline, or a combination of both techniques. The surgical approach is determined by where in the spine the tumor is located, the cervical spine, the thoracic spine, the lumbar spine, or the sacrum; what specific bone it's in, whether in the front of the spinal column or behind the spinal canal; and the extent of the involvement, whether it involves just one vertebral body or multiple sites. It is difficult to operate around the spinal cord. A surgeon usually will not approach the tumor in the cervical or thoracic spine posteriorly when the spinal cord is intimately involved because the spinal cord can't be retracted (moved around) without paralyzing the patient.

The major problem with metastatic diseases is that cancer is now a systemic problem. Someone who has breast cancer or lung cancer that spreads to the spine, by definition, has cancer throughout the body; the issue is no longer curing the disease but controlling it. Surgeons are, in that instance, just one member of the team of doctors, and their role is to control the local disease specific to the spine and to work along with medical oncologists, radiation therapists, and the patient's internist—the primary care providers for the global treatment of metastatic disease.

We need to say a few words about treatment that is specifically available for a disease called *myeloma*, which originates from the bone marrow cell and leads to a weakening of the bone throughout the body and also commonly affects the spinal column. Occasionally, myeloma can lead to significant compression fractures, just as we see in people with osteoporosis. The fractures may impair sexual function as well as bladder and bowel function and cause weakness or complete paralysis in the limbs. In addition to receiving steroids and other chemotherapy agents, people with this type of cancer are often treated with vertebroplasty and kyphoplasty procedures, which are very effective in treating the pain related to vertebral body collapse. (These treatments are described in Chapter 6.) Just as they do in people with osteoporosis, the multiple compression fractures cause the person to become shorter over time. In terms of how the spinal column looks, a young person in his or her forties may resemble someone in his or her eighties. Myeloma is sensitive to radiation therapy, and for the most part, people with this cancer respond well to radiation and chemotherapy.

Cancer treatment designed to prolong and save lives can cause long-term problems, such as memory loss and neuropathy and, significantly, can also cause other cancers. Whenever a patient is diagnosed with a tumor in an area that has received radiation treatment in the past, we are extremely uncomfortable because radiation in the long run can cause a cancer called *radiation-induced sarcoma*. Usually, these tumors have a bad prognosis.

Primary Tumors of the Spine

If a young person has a tumor, it's more likely to be a primary tumor than metastatic disease. Primary tumors of the spine are rare tumors that begin in the bone, cartilage, or other tissues in and around the spine. The nerves, the spinal cord, and the covering of nerves, all located inside the spinal column, can be a source of tumor growth. These tumors range in their behavior from fairly benign tumors to very aggressive tumors. These tumors affect different parts of the vertebra. The tumors that affect the dorsal (back) part of the spinal column in younger patients tend to be benign, and the tumors that affect the vertebral bodies—the front part of the spinal column—are more often malignant. Just like some metastatic tumors, some of these tumors are extremely vascular—they contain many blood vessels—and they need to be embolized before surgery.

Some tumors, such as chordoma or chondrosarcoma, do not respond to chemotherapy or radiation therapy. The best treatment option for these tumors is complete removal of the tumor. In other situations, such as with a tumor-like bone cyst called the *aneurysmal* bone cyst, the tumor is relatively benign and can be treated by cleaning up the inside of the tumor and packing the area with bone. Complete removal is not necessary for controlling this relatively benign tumor. (*Relatively benign* means that the tumor does not go to other parts of the body, and locally, the risk of the tumor recurring is relatively low, even when a tumor is treated in a way that leaves something behind.)

When we look at tumors, we consider the following:

- How fast will it grow?
- What is the likelihood of it spreading to other parts of the body?
- Where is it?
- What techniques can be used to either kill it or slow it down?

The answers to these questions are used to decide how to treat the tumor. When a person has an abnormality in the spinal column, it may look like a tumor. First, we take images, including CT, MRI scans, and plain x-rays. Then we obtain a biopsy (placing a needle in the tumor to obtain a tissue sample) and perform other tests (laboratory blood tests, for example). These tests, the person's age, and the location in the spine provide clues about what is going on, and we base treatment on this information. If it is a primary tumor and it appears to be coming from the spine but has spread all over the body, it would probably not be addressed surgically.

If it has not spread, we would probably try to remove the tumor and cure the patient. We perform surgery and, if needed, add chemotherapy and radiation treatment to give the person the best chance of being cured. Osteogenic sarcoma occasionally arises from the spinal column or sacrum, and it has a high potential to spread to other parts of the body, such as the lungs. The treatment of this tumor requires all the weapons we have: chemotherapy, surgery, more chemotherapy, and potentially radiotherapy. This is the only way to control the tumor both locally and systemically.

Back Pain at a Glance: What Are the Warning Signs of Tumors?
We do not want to unduly alarm you by describing the warning signs of cancer, so we begin by saying that many conditions besides cancer cause pain. More than 90 percent of the time back pain is not a sign of a primary or metastatic spinal tumor but is instead an indication of a common condition, such as muscle strain and degenerative disc disease. However, see your physician if you are over 50 years old and you exhibit the following symptoms:
- Constant night pain
- Pain with no history of trauma
- Pain unrelated to activity
- Unexplained weight loss
- A personal history of cancer

Types of Spinal Cord Tumors

So far we have discussed the tumors that originate outside the sac (dura) in which the spinal cord is located. In this section, we review the tumors that arise within the dura. These include tumors growing within the substance of the spinal cord (intramedullary tumors) and those that form outside the spinal cord, originating from the nerves (nerve sheath tumors) and membranes (meningioma).

Tumors called *nerve sheath tumors* originate in the nerves. They are usually benign and can be excised completely, and most patients are cured of disease. With a nerve sheath tumor, a nerve goes into the tumor and a nerve comes out of the tumor. The surgeon must make sure that the nerve is not functionally critical to the patient. Fortunately, it usually is not. To make sure of this, before the surgery, the surgeon places needles in the patient's legs and various muscles to which electrical impulses from the nerves in this area travel. The surgeon also places needles in the anal sphincter and connects leads to an EMG machine, which records the activity of the muscle. Then, during the surgery, special electrical probes are put on the nerves, electrical stimulation is applied, and electrical activity from the muscles is recorded. The information this process provides allows the surgeon to decide whether a nerve is functionally critical. Responses from the legs are recorded, and if we find that the nerve is not doing anything significant (typically, it is just providing sensation), it can be cut above and below the nerve sheath without danger of impairing the patient's ability to function.

Another type of tumor in this area is *meningioma*, which is a common tumor that originates in the covering of the spinal cord called *meninges*. These tumors, too, are mostly benign and can be excised in most situations, and the patient is usually cured. The surgeon usually can debulk (remove in pieces) nerve sheath tumors and meningiomas, making them smaller and easier to remove.

The situation is different with a special form of *ependymoma* (called a *myxopapillary ependymoma*), a type of tumor that originates from the spinal cord. Debulking is not appropriate for this type of tumor. The tumor should be excised completely in one piece, and if the surgery goes well, the patient is cured. However, if cancer cells from this type of ependymoma are spilled into cerebral spinal fluid during surgery, it becomes an incurable condition despite additional treatment such as radiation therapy. To prevent this situation, the surgeon must realize that the tumor is a myxopapillary ependymoma and must try to remove it in one piece, without entering the tumor.

Should someone with a primary spinal cord tumor seek the attention of a specialist surgeon, such as a neuro-oncologist or an oncological neurosurgeon? It takes experience and skill to identify and to remove a tumor such as an ependymoma, and we have discussed why it is essential for this surgery to be performed with great care. Ependymomas are commonly misleading in appearance, and they are difficult to differentiate from nerve sheath tumors. With experience, the surgeon is prepared. When a surgeon removes a tumor that may or may not be an ependymoma, the surgeon should treat it as if it is. Having explained why we recommend that you are seen by an experienced specialist surgeon, we must also say that if you have *sudden onset of paralysis or weakness*, you may not have time to see a specialist (see the box titled "When Is It an Emergency?"). Most of the time when someone comes in feeling weak, we order an MRI or CT scan of that area, which will show the tumor, and we relieve pressure on the spinal cord as quickly as possible. If someone is weak, we can reverse it most of the time, but if they are paralyzed, by the time they come in for treatment, it may be too late. When someone is paralyzed, quick diagnosis and treatment are crucial.

Another group of malignant tumors originating from the spinal cord is called *astrocytomas*. Highly malignant variants of these tumors usually cannot be cured with surgery and require additional treatment such as radiation.

Treating Cancer

When we treat cancer in any part of the body, we have two goals in mind: (1) to eradicate the tumor or control the tumor locally where it has originated and (2) if the tumor has already spread to other spots in the body beyond its original site, then we try to control that spread and treat the cancer in other parts of the body. At this time, we have only three general treatment options: (1) surgery, which involves resecting (cutting) something out; (2) radiation therapy, which involves drawing a target and then firing a bunch of bullets at that target, using a radiation beam; and (3) chemotherapy, which will be administered orally or by IV as a means to kill the tumor in areas away from the original site. Chemotherapy is a systemic killing, or remote killing, of the tumor all throughout the body.

For every person who has cancer, we try to determine whether the disease is local or whether it has spread to other parts of the body. If the disease is local, the primary goal is to try to control it locally—cut it out and maybe give it additional radiation therapy, which is a local treatment. We cannot radiate the entire body, so if the patient already has distant spots (if there is metastatic disease), then we have to have a treatment that will control the tumor outside of the primary site. This treatment is chemotherapy, which travels through the bloodstream all over the body.

Based on the type of tumor, we know how likely it is to remain local and the metastatic potential of the tumor, if it has not already metastasized. Consider a woman with breast cancer who has a lumpectomy (removal of the tumor from the breast) and a sampling of lymph nodes in the armpit: If the tumor was removed from the primary site of the breast completely but the patient had a number of lymph nodes that were positive for tumor, the physician would obtain a chest x-ray, an abdominal CT scan, and other studies to look at the rest of the body. If these tests are negative, the tumor, as far as we can tell, has not spread to other parts of the body. In this situation, the tumor has been cut out locally, but because the patient's disease has already spread to the lymph nodes in the armpit (which is near the site of the original tumor), the chances of the patient having disease elsewhere are rather high, despite the results of the imaging tests. In this situation, additional radiation to that area and chemotherapy might be prescribed. Because we know that the patient is likely to develop the disease elsewhere, or the disease might already be elsewhere and so small that we cannot detect it, treating it is the wise thing to do.

Radiation works by killing the dividing cells. In fact, it kills every dividing cell when the radiation is given, including healthy cells. Since tumor cells divide more rapidly and more of the populations of cells are dividing at one time, it kills more of the tumor cells than the normal tissue; it is said to semi-selectively kill the tumor cells. With traditional or conventional radiation, a dose of radiation is spread out over days to an area that includes the tumor and normal structures around it. (Stereotactic radiation, described previously, is different from traditional or conventional radiation.) Radiation has an effect on the normal structures just as it has on the tumor but to a lesser degree because the other cells are not dividing as rapidly and have greater capacity to heal themselves from radiation damage than the cancer cells do. What limits the dosage of radiation we are able to give depends on the dose normal tissues around the tumor will tolerate and the dose beyond that which is harmful to those tissues. The balance is to avoid giving the harmful dose to the spinal cord, to the intestines, or to the normal structures, while giving enough radiation to kill all or most of the remaining tumor cells.

In conventional radiation, we draw a box around the tumor—a rectangular box most of the time—and use two different ports (sites of entry) to administer the radiation, one from front to back and one from side to side. The radiologist who is giving the treatment essentially "hits" everything in the box; unfortunately, the shape of the box does not necessarily fit the shape of the tumor. We give

Back Pain at a Glance: What Are the Promising New Treatments for Spinal Tumors?

- Stereotactic radiosurgery
- Genetically engineered therapies
- Targeted drugs such as angiostatin

half of the radiation from one angle and half of the radiation from another angle so the tissues around the tumors, although they receive a lot of radiation, receive less than they would if we were to direct the entire radiation dose at one point. Still, there is significant radiation to normal tissue. The dose has to be high enough to kill the tumor but low enough that the tissue around the tumor is not significantly damaged.

With the conventional method of radiation treatment, we can administer radiation through two or possibly three different ports, and that's it. We divide the dose into two or three different fragments and then the target will get the total amount of radiation in two directions, and normal tissue surrounding the target will get only half or one-third of the dose.

The recent advance in the use of radiation is a technique called *stereotactic radiosurgery*. In this treatment, instead of a single beam of radiation directed at an area, there are multiple small beams coming from different directions, and these small beams at a lower dose intersect at the location of the tumor. The multiple small doses add up to a lethal dose just in the tumor itself. Instead of just having two or three different portals of entry for the radiation, there are maybe 250 to 300 different trajectories. Say, we are targeting the center of a soccer ball and that we shine lights from 500 different sources at the ball; all of these lights go through the surface of the ball and come together in the center of the ball. On the surface of the sphere, you get one light shining in one spot, but in the center of the sphere, all of these lights come together, so the target in the middle is hit by all of the lights. With stereotactic radiosurgery, we can increase the dose but with less effect on the normal tissues around the spine.

Before we perform stereotactic radiosurgery, we must obtain CT and MRI scans. Sometimes we place markers around the tumor and take other steps to get an accurate idea of the location and shape of the tumor for radiation therapy. We may implant markers made out of gold or other metals at the time of surgery, or we may use an implant that is put in at the time of the surgery. For someone who hasn't previously had surgery for the disease, a surgical procedure is sometimes done to implant markers, but some of the newer stereotactic radiosurgeries don't need markers and can be guided by CT scans.

Stereotactic surgery has been in common use for the past ten years and has been available in most major cancer centers for the past five years. As the computer technology and imaging technology has improved and become more precise, automated, and cheaper, the technique has become more widespread. Ten years ago, there were two centers in the country that administered stereotactic treatment using proton beam radiation: Boston, Massachusetts, and Loma Linda, California. The first common spine application was with the cyberknife, which was first used in Stanford University. In Baltimore, three centers now perform stereotactic radiosurgery, each one with a slightly different approach.

When a new treatment is not available everywhere in the country, we must consider whether the outcomes are so significantly different that a person should travel to a center that uses this method. In some instances, stereotactic radiosurgery improves outcome or may even prevent the need for surgery. In other instances, if someone already has had radiation or has had nearly a lethal dose or a dangerous dose to the spinal cord, the intestines, or other structures, the stereotactic approach will allow retreatment, spot treatment, or touch-up treatment in the area. When the type of tumor is not likely to spread to other locations or beyond where it can be seen on imaging studies, stereotactic radiosurgery can replace an operation. So, it has some advantages over conventional therapy in some cases.

Your doctor may tell you that this new approach is not advantageous to you, and there are times when conventional radiation is actually a benefit. Conventional therapy is a benefit when we try to treat the region around the area the tumor occupies. Sometimes we know exactly where to treat, but if we don't, then conventional radiation is as effective as, and may be more effective than, the stereotactic approach. If the margins of the tumor are not entirely clear, and if there is a chance for the tumor to be located beyond where we can see it on scans, then drawing a box and radiating everything inside the box is better than stereotactic radiosurgery. (If the margins are precise and there is a critical structure next to the tumor, such as the spinal cord, then stereotactic radiosurgery absolutely has a benefit.) If you are offered standard radiation treatment, it does not mean that your outlook is poorer.

Cancer treatment requires a team approach, so physicians, surgeons, radiation therapists, oncologists (chemotherapists), and the internist work together to decide on the timing and the best course of treatment. Timing of the elements of treatment—surgery, radiation therapy, and chemotherapy—is critical. After surgery, for example, there is often a specific waiting period before radiation and chemotherapy can begin or resume. Radiation and chemotherapy prevent healing of the surgical incision, so we must allow the skin and soft tissues to heal before these other treatments are given. Usually, if an operation is warranted, it's better to have the operation before radiation rather than after radiation. Surgery can be performed after radiation, but the risks are higher in terms of wound healing, leakage of the spinal fluid, and wound breakdown. The treatment team will work together to decide whether you have radiation and chemotherapy before the surgery (or even during the surgery), how it is delivered, and then how long to wait until after the surgery before starting other treatments.

When we perform surgery for metastatic disease, we are trying to decrease people's pain, maintain and increase their mobility, and prevent paralysis, or, if they have some neurological impairment, then we are trying to reverse or minimize it. We try to do the surgery in a way that minimizes patients' hospital stay and allows them to receive continued radiation and chemotherapy treatment of their metastatic disease.

Patients with metastatic spine disease have the disease elsewhere in the body—in the lungs, liver, and other organs. These patients have multiple areas in their spinal column, and the disease is causing spinal cord compression, paralysis, and excruciating pain. Sometimes the disease is so extensive that patients are not healthy enough to undergo general anesthesia for a major surgical procedure. Unfortunately, we must tell them that they are too sick for surgery. Again, we are tying to improve the person's quality of life, and early death from complications of surgery does not accomplish that. We must make these difficult decisions based on the extent of patients' disability, what we will need to do to address that, and, if it can be addressed with surgery, how long the recovery will take.

A tumor grows by dividing, and as it divides it secretes vascular growth factor (VGF) to get more nutrients. VGF is a special chemical that the tumor cells put out so that they can stimulate the blood vessels around the tumor to branch out and try to feed this new growth. Researchers recently discovered an anti-VGF substance called *angiostatin*. These researchers demonstrated that when mice were given the medication, although the tumor continued to grow, it could not acquire the blood vessels to sustain its growth and the tumor eventually died. Although angiostatin is one of the strategies used to treat tumors, particularly vascular tumors, in humans, it is used only on a trial basis. Sadly, we have cured cancer in mice many times in the past without successfully transferring the cure to humans. The difficulty (and the delight) of being human is that higher mammals have a complicated set of pathways to the human cells, and the pathways circumvent the barrier erected in front of the tumor growth.

Significant advances have been made in cancer treatment in the past decade, some of them within the past five years. Now we have a better understanding of how cancer cells grow, what makes them grow, and what makes them stop growing. A future strategy will probably involve multiple sites of targets in a human cell. With current chemotherapy and radiation therapy, we injure or kill normal cells along with cancer cells. The challenge comes when we try to be selective; what we really want to do is selectively attack cells at multiple levels.

The trend is to operate on people with advanced disease more often now than five or ten years ago because chemotherapy, radiation, and other nonsurgical techniques have improved significantly; therefore, disease is being controlled better. We are seeing more patients with spinal involvement and with more advanced disease because people live longer. We often make decisions to operate because people are living longer and are in better shape than they would have been before recent advances in treatment. Their prognosis for living longer is better. We can do many things for them, not necessarily surgically but medically—radiation therapy, for example. Real advances have been made, and the treatment of cancer is much more successful than before.

Back Pain at a Glance: When Is It an Emergency?

Someone with a primary or metastatic tumor whose only symptom is pain or mild weakness has the option of seeking advice and treatment from surgical experts—someone who does this surgery all the time. But there are instances in which there is no time for delay. In the following situations, seek medical attention immediately:

- Sudden paralysis
- Sudden weakness
- Sudden loss of bowel or bladder control

When someone has paralysis or sudden loss of spinal cord function, this is an emergency and needs to be immediately addressed. If you are suddenly weak or suddenly paralyzed and you have prompt surgery—within several hours—your chances of recovery are greater. After complete paralysis lasts more than twelve hours, the chances of recovering full function decrease significantly. A limited emergency operation can be performed to relieve pressure on the spinal cord, and then afterward the patient can seek other opinions about other surgery.

Treating Cancer Pain

Pain is complicated and involves different structures in a complex way. There are surgeries and other techniques for blocking pain, but pain is hard to turn off. When the pain is due to cancer, it can be especially difficult to control.

We can administer narcotic pain medicines directly into the spinal canal to try to reduce the systemic side effects of pain medications. This procedure increases the medications' central effects on the nerves. We can also put in electrodes and other things to direct a current around nerves and try to block them. We know that if we block the nerves before they actually carry pain sensation to the brain, we can reduce someone's perception of pain and their response to painful stimuli. We do that often in surgery by giving local numbing medications (that essentially block pain) to people before we cut the skin, even though the patients are already sedated (see Chapter 9). After surgery, we give them other medicines that block or reduce the pain before they experience pain.

Cutting nerves usually is not a long-term solution or effective treatment for pain because even though the nerve has been cut and no signals are coming from it (or even if we cut the spinal cord where signals are being carried to the brain), the brain can still feel the pain. We don't quite understand why that happens, but probably the signals are carried by other nerves in the vicinity of the spinal cord, or some blocking nerve fibers are cut, so signals are electrically sent in a way that gets the pain message through, even though there are no signals coming in. The situation is similar to phantom limb pain in which even after amputation, the brain still feels the leg or an arm in place.

One surgical treatment for cancer pain is *rhizotomy*, an operation that involves exposing the specific nerve carrying the pain signal. As we described in Chapter 1, the nerve has two components to it as it comes out of the spinal cord. One component carries the sensory signal, and the other carries the motor signal. In a rhizotomy, the surgeon identifies the two components of the nerves and cuts only the ones that carry the sensory signals. This operation can effectively diminish or eliminate the pain in a given spot, but unfortunately, the benefits of cutting the sensory nerve do not last long. Usually, after about a year, the individual gets similar pain.

Pain is a difficult condition to treat. Fortunately, recent advances in medicine have led to the development of devices such as morphine pumps, spinal cord stimulators, and a new set of surgical procedures (such as deep brain stimulation), making it possible for physicians to more effectively address this debilitating condition.

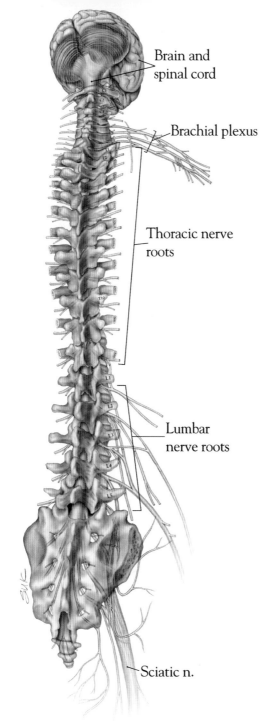

Brain and
spinal cord

Brachial plexus

Thoracic nerve
roots

Lumbar
nerve roots

Sciatic n.

Figure 1. The spine. Nerves emanate from the spinal cord transmit signals from the brain to the body and from the body to the brain.

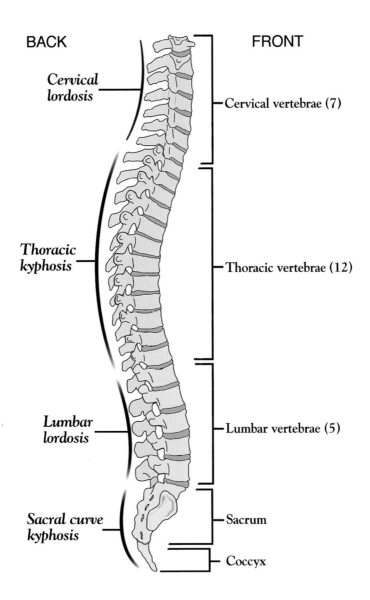

BACK   FRONT

Cervical
lordosis   — Cervical vertebrae (7)

Thoracic
kyphosis   — Thoracic vertebrae (12)

Lumbar
lordosis   — Lumbar vertebrae (5)

Sacral curve
kyphosis   — Sacrum

                                        — Coccyx

Figure 2. The regions of the spine. The primary regions of the spine are
(1) the *cervical spine* (the neck), with 7 vertebrae, (2) the *thoracic spine* (the chest
region, or the middle of the back), with 12 vertebrae, (3) the *lumbar spine* (the
lower back), with 5 vertebrae, (4) and the *sacrum*. Located below the sacrum is
the very small "tail" bone called the *coccyx*. These regions also provide the four
curves in the back, illustrated on the left side of the illustration.

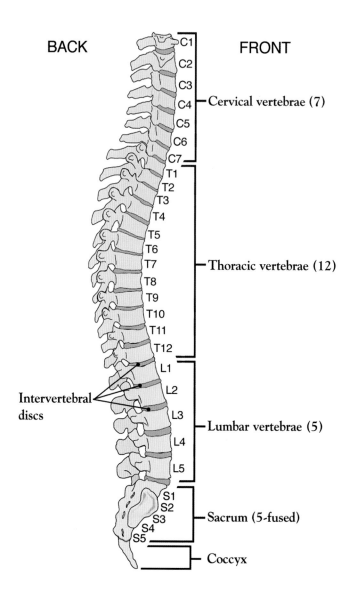

BACK

FRONT

C1
C2
C3
C4 — Cervical vertebrae (7)
C5
C6
C7

T1
T2
T3
T4
T5
T6
T7 — Thoracic vertebrae (12)
T8
T9
T10
T11
T12

Intervertebral discs

L1
L2
L3 — Lumbar vertebrae (5)
L4
L5

S1
S2
S3 — Sacrum (5-fused)
S4
S5

Coccyx

Figure 3. The numbered vertebrae. The vertebrae are numbered C1 through C7, T1 through T12, L1 through L5, S1 through S5. The numbering begins at the top of each region.

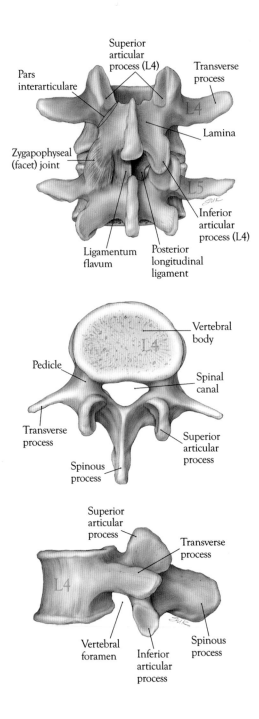

Figure 4. Close-up of a vertebra from the back, the top, and the side.

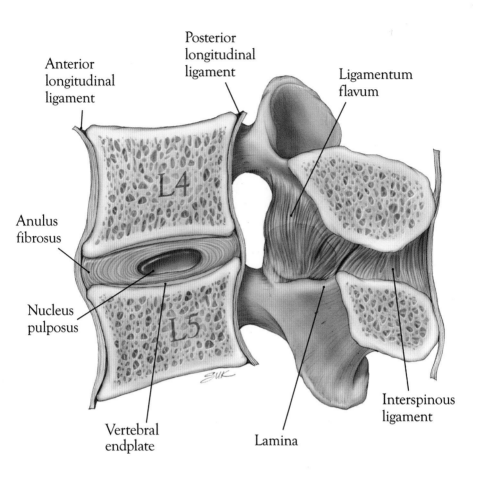

Figure 5. Inside a vertebra. A cut through the middle from front to back at L4 and L5 vertebrae level (side view), showing the intervertebral disk.

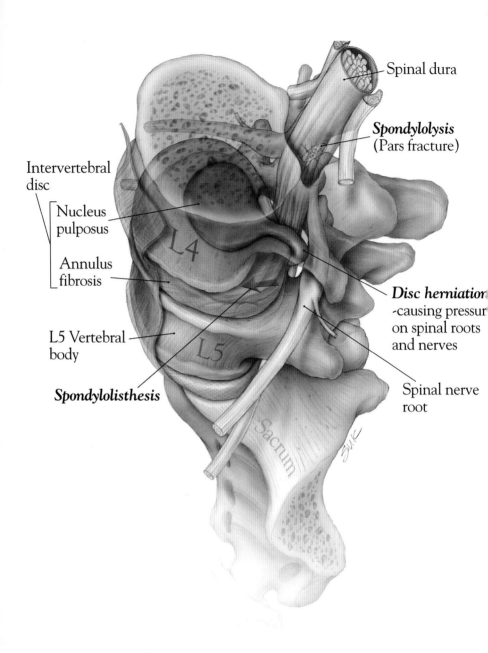

Spinal dura

Spondylolysis
(Pars fracture)

Intervertebral
disc

Nucleus
pulposus

Annulus
fibrosis

L4

L5

L5 Vertebral
body

Disc herniation
-causing pressure
on spinal roots
and nerves

Spinal nerve
root

Spondylolisthesis

Sacrum

Figure 6. Close-up of disc herniation, spondylolysis, and spondylolisthesis.

Figure 7 (facing page). Full view of lordosis, kyphosis, spondylolysis, and
spondylolisthesis.

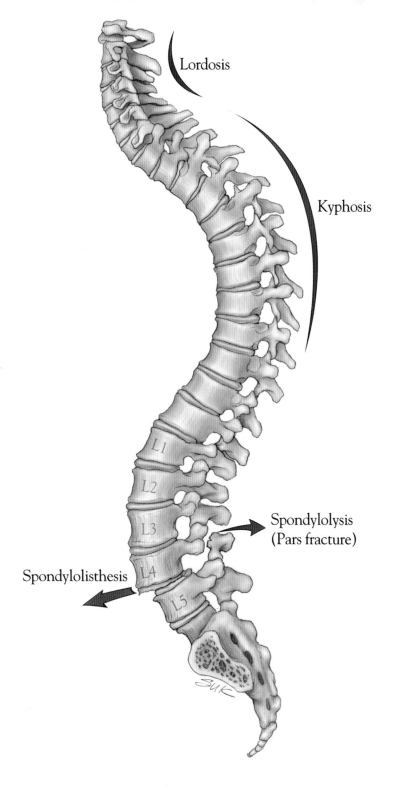

Lordosis

Kyphosis

L1

L2

L3

Spondylolysis
(Pars fracture)

L4

Spondylolisthesis

L5

SUK

Part II
Getting a Diagnosis and Seeking Treatment

Five

What's Wrong with Me, and What Should I Do about It?

WHEN YOU ASK A doctor, "What would you do if this was your back?" the doctor may not have a clear answer because many times there is not a single right solution to the problem. Some problems have a clear solution that most doctors would agree on. In other instances, there is no right or wrong choice. The patient who has a tumor or cancer metastasis, for example, needs immediate treatment. However, when a person experiences pain without a definite cause, the right treatment is less obvious. Pain is a subjective complaint, and no one can know how much pain someone else is in. Different people are willing or able to tolerate different amounts of pain. Attitudes toward taking medications, having surgery, and activity modification vary from individual to individual. Most of the time, then, what a doctor would do in the context of his or her own life and circumstance may not help in clarifying what you should do. It is largely up to you to answer the question based on how you address the problem, the pain, and your expectations.

Studies have shown that most back pain improves within two months from the time it begins, with or without treatment. This means that delaying surgery for back pain is usually a sound option! As we'll see in Chapter 6, pain and discomfort can be relieved in many ways as the natural healing process takes place. Because of the variety of approaches for treating spinal conditions, it is especially important for you to be informed and to participate in decisions about your medical care.

The doctor can tell the patient who has a specific problem that a certain procedure makes sense for some patients in his or her situation. But even among doctors, the approach to surgery differs. For a person with lumbar disc disease, one doctor might recommend artificial disc surgery, while another might recommend fusion surgery. A third might recommend no surgery at all. Different recommendations arise because expertise, training, and philosophies differ among surgeons and because we just don't know as much about the cause of back pain and treatment outcomes as we'd like.

In Chapter 6, we describe nonsurgical approaches to treating back problems; in Chapter 8, we explain the factors to consider when deciding to have surgery; and in Chapter 9, we focus on back surgery and recovery. Whether surgical or nonsurgical, the best treatment for a specific individual depends on the diagnosis and the person's expectations. After discussing the various sources of medical information you will encounter, we turn in this chapter to exploring the route to diagnosis—including how diagnostic tests are done and what they show and don't show as well as a few words about the doctor-patient relationship—which leads to making a decision about what treatment is right for you.

The World of Medical Information

Many patients who visit their doctor have already read about their condition on the Internet or in a book like this one, and they are seeking their doctor's opinion about what choice they should make among the options they have already read or heard about. Information about the back is all around us: There is information in the lay press, information provided by friends and relatives, information provided on the Internet, and information provided by health care professionals.

To some degree, all of these resources are potentially useful; however, different weights must be assigned to different sources of information. Why? Because information undergoes varying degrees of filtering, depending on the source, and the Internet is the most unfiltered. On the Internet, you put a specific word or a series of words into a search engine, and you get information from an array of sources, some reputable, some not.

The most respectable Internet sources about the spine are those sites maintained by spine societies or subspecialty societies. You can get all kinds of information from Europe, South America, Asia, the former Communist bloc, the Middle East, or Africa, but the most relevant to the American public are English-language sites from subspecialty spine societies. Most of these web sites have patient-oriented pages, and the posted information goes through an author and topic review process. Then the information is edited for appropriateness for the public. These sites are sophisticated, up to date, and express a consensus view. That is, they tend to avoid the extremes of aggressive or conservative. They discuss newer technologies as well, and put them within the context of older, more proven technologies.

We recommend these web sites:

- American Academy of Orthopedic Surgeons, www.aaos.org
- American Association of Neurological Surgeons, www.aans.org
- Cervical Spine Research Society, www.csrs.org
- Congress of Neurological Surgeons, www.neurosurgeon.org
- North American Spine Society, www.spine.org
- Scoliosis Research Society, www.srs.org

Your surgeon is probably familiar with these web sites or, at least aware of them, because these sites often include information that is presented, taught, and discussed among surgeons. If you are familiar with the sites, too, then you and your physician can use the information from the web site as common ground for a discussion.

That said, if you start your encounter with your physician by asking her or him about a web page or a specific treatment, you are not getting the most out of your doctor visit. You are better off asking those questions after you have given the doctor an opportunity to do what doctors do best, and what you are primarily there for, which is to get their opinion of what they think is wrong and what they think would be the best treatment for you. If you are seeing the doctor to ask about a web page or about a new study that you heard about on the radio, you probably can't expect your doctor to devote as much time and effort to the task of determining what she thinks is wrong with you and what treatment to recommend. If your information comes from a web site, a television show, or a newspaper, your doctor cannot be expected to be an expert on that particular topic; it's possible that the story is so recent that your doctor won't have much more information about it than you do.

Use your doctors as a resource. First, allow them to go through the process of diagnosing your symptoms and recommending the best treatment options, based on their own experience and knowledge. After they have done their job, you might ask them what they think about a specific treatment you've heard or read about.

With the Internet, there is often no filter and no accountability, which makes it unreliable and sometimes even dangerous. You will want to identify online sources associated with credible and accountable organizations whose reputations are based solely on providing information about the spine or the back. These organizations do not have an agenda, such as selling a health product, as some online sources do. Use the Internet with caution.

There is absolutely no accountability in chat rooms. People participating in the chat room can say whatever they want to say and claim to be whoever they want to be, and there are no repercussions. You don't know whether they are lying or even whether five of the people with different names in the chat room are all the same person. Read and participate in chat rooms with caution.

Company web sites can be useful, but they, too, can have an agenda. They often are the only information source for new and emerging technologies and treatments (for example, company web sites recently provided some of the first and most complete information about artificial disc replacements). But they are not going to give you a balanced view. Companies can provide you with the name of a surgeon who can provide their service (or use their technology), but they will not make any judgment about the surgeons' abilities. Keep in mind that you are reading information provided by a commercial entity.

If you are deciding whether you should begin to take a medication, it can be intimidating to read the warning label and the laundry list of side effects. By federal regulation, drug companies must list side effects of their products on their package label, but they don't necessarily list their frequency or severity. If you are *experiencing* a side effect, look at the package label to find out whether it is a side effect associated with that particular drug. A person who is concerned about such things may be overwhelmed by the possibility of the many side effects that are listed. It is probably reasonable to read about the possible side effects if you are concerned, but be sure to ask your doctor whether he or she believes that it is reasonable for you to take the medication. He or she will have a greater perspective than can be gained by just reading the warning label and will put the information into context for you, taking into account the risk/benefit ratio of this medication specifically for you.

Sometimes a news story will be released in the press before the information has been disseminated to the medical community. Articles in the press can be useful, but they may not be balanced. Many writers, reporters, and others who provide information through the popular media have limited knowledge and limited time to acquire the depth of knowledge needed to present medical topics. Information tends to be superficial and often fails to put stories in a broader context because of the time constraints and a limited understanding of the issues. These news outlets serve a purpose for alerting people to new trends and ideas, but remember that the newer a treatment is, the less likely *anyone* will be able to put it into a broader context or even have a record or experience with the treatment.

Friends, neighbors, relatives, and co-workers will be able to tell you whether they had a good experience with a specific doctor, whether the doctor was someone they liked or disliked, trusted or mistrusted, and whether the doctor seemed generally reasonable. If they did not like the doctor and did not trust him and could substantiate their feelings, then you can probably consider their information to be valid. However, you might get along just fine with that same doctor. Can medical information or experiences specific to other people be translated directly to your case? Many people, in trying to be helpful, offer information and describe experiences they have had, but that information and those experiences may not be relative to your specific condition.

What about books? You will want to know whether the author's goal is to provide options and broad information on many topics or to push a specific agenda. For a general book on back pain, we recommend *Maggie's Back Book: Healing the Hurt in Your Lower Back*, by Margaret B. Lettvin, which was published about thirty years ago and still holds true.

Information about Your Problem

The most useful source of information for you is your family doctor. That's probably where you want to start. For one thing, you and your family doctor (or internist) know each other. Furthermore, back pain often is something the family doctor and internist can treat. If they can't help you, they will know specialists you can see, and they can point you in the right direction. Nonmedical people such as friends and family are not the best source of information. They don't have the medical background to make an educated

Back Pain at a Glance: What Do Pain Scales Tell Doctors about My Pain?
Your doctor's office probably has asked you the question a dozen times: "On a scale of one to ten, how bad is your pain today?" The pain scales used in medicine today came about when health care professionals became aware that they may not always have addressed patients' pain symptoms as well as they might have (partly because they were focused on finding the *cause* of the pain as a way of relieving the pain in the long term). These scales tell us how a specific patient is *experiencing* pain, but they don't tell us much about how bad the pain actually is.

There is no way to measure pain objectively; we can only appreciate the patient's subjective experience of pain. We can't always tell which patients simply tolerate a higher level of pain and which patients can't tolerate much pain at all. Thus, someone may have a serious problem but may report having only minimal pain, while someone else with nothing much wrong may be nearly incapacitated by pain. By making this observation, we are not judging anyone. Pain is an important symptom and it needs to be paid attention to. It is a fact, however, that different people experience pain differently.

guess about your problem, and most of the time they don't have access to your individual medical history. (You probably don't want your neighbor knowing all your medical history, anyway!)

Diagnostic Tests

The diagnostic tests described here are used to diagnose both acute and chronic back pain, though most people with acute back pain find that the pain goes away on its own after a relatively brief time, while a person with chronic back pain is more likely to seek medical attention and seek it repeatedly. Physicians more often find it necessary to perform diagnostic tests to identify the cause of chronic pain, as well.

If you are scheduled to have a diagnostic test, you will receive instructions in person or by telephone from your doctor and possibly also from someone in the office where the test will be performed. You may be given a printed instructional booklet. Although the tests are performed more or less the same in different settings, there may be slight variations. You need to follow the instructions you are given by your own doctor or other health care professional.

Imaging Tests

Imaging tests are the first line of tests for diagnosing the cause of back pain. They are useful and generally safe. Pregnant women or women who may be pregnant should not be exposed to x-rays or have a CT scan, except under special circumstances, although an MRI scan is considered safe.

Imaging tests may involve an injection of contrast material, or dye, to which some people have an allergic reaction. If you know you have an allergy to radiologic dyes or iodine, let your doctor know before the test. If you itch, have shortness of breath, or develop hives after the injection of dye, tell the technician administering the test so you can be monitored and given medications if necessary.

X-rays

X-rays are what we have referred to in these pages as plain x-ray. They are taken by standard x-ray machines, often during your visit with your doctor. X-rays can show arthritis, fractures, infections, and tumors and are useful in defining the overall shape, alignment, and motion in the back.

Computed Tomography

Computed tomography (called CT scan or CAT scan) is an advanced x-ray technology that provides detailed images of the body. A thin beam of x-rays is directed at the body and then a computer takes the information provided by the x-rays and composes a detailed picture of the body part or area. The CT image is more detailed than a standard x-ray, showing, for example, not just the skull bones but also the brain within the skull. A three-dimensional CT scan can be obtained by using a special computer to process information from the regular CT scan.

You may receive an injection of dye ("contrast"), which helps define any abnormalities. You lie perfectly still on the scanning table as the table moves to position you within the doughnut-shaped hole in the scanner. A CT scan lasts less than one minute to up to one hour for a myelogram CT scan.

To MRI or Not to MRI

Magnetic resonance imaging (MRI) is a form of diagnostic imaging that uses strong magnets to produce cross-section images of structures within the body. Having an MRI involves lying on a table rolled into the MRI machine; again, you lie perfectly still while the MRI machine takes images. The machine makes loud banging noises while it is in use, so patients sometimes wear headphones or earplugs during the test. It can be claustrophobic as well as noisy inside the MRI machine, and some people find it more comfortable if they wear a blindfold or eye covers so they can't see the tunnel while they are inside. MRI is not safe for people with some pacemakers and some metal implants or objects in their bodies.

MRI scans play an important role in diagnosing back problems, as you can tell by the number of times the test has been mentioned in these pages. But we want to emphasize that an MRI scan may fail to identify the source of the problem, and it may also mislead both the patient and the physician down the wrong route to treatment.

In one MRI study, people who had never had back pain were used as normal controls. When scans were done, it was found that even people who did not have back pain had findings on the MRI that showed that the spine was not perfect. The reality is that imaging studies reflect the normal aging process and that most of the changes seen on an x-ray or MRI scans tend not to be relevant to your symptoms. Furthermore, when a study is obtained, it is usually obtained to answer a specific question, and answering that specific question is really the purpose of the study. The purpose of the study is not to see all the things that are wrong with your back, because many of the things that are not normal with your back that the study can detect are things that do not cause pain or symptoms. For example, finding a bulging disc on an MRI scan can be of little or no relevance to your symptoms.

Physicians order tests because they are trying to answer specific questions. In someone who has had back pain for a couple of months with no known cause, the physician asks, "Does this patient have a tumor? Infection? Fracture?" This question is more useful than, "Does this patient have arthritis?" because we expect to see arthritic changes in a person in his or her forties or fifties, and what we are trying *not* to do is miss another cause of back pain, such as a tumor or infection. Arthritis detected on a plain x-ray or MRI scan in someone in his forties or fifties is normal. We are looking for the abnormal.

MRI scans are probably one of the most overprescribed tests performed for back pain. A doctor often orders an MRI for back pain when taking a plain x-ray or just waiting for the back pain to ease would be sufficient. Many physicians who order the MRI do not know its purpose or do not know the natural history studies (showing that most people get better from back pain on their own). What happens next is that a person with a bulging disc and loss of water content in the disc or stenosis—all the things that radiologists read on the scan—worries. The first physician sends the patient to a specialist to interpret the x-ray and MRI scan, and the specialist tells the patient not to worry—this is not a problem. The patient is anxious by the time he sees the specialist; however, and his expectation is that he has a problem that the specialist will address. The specialist must explain that the MRI scan is not a good test to solve this problem or to provide any relief, information, or insight about the cause of the problem. Most people can *see* the changes; they just do not *understand* them. A specialist spends time explaining test results that are not perfect but are within the normal range for most people.

CT Myelogram

If the MRI does not show the problem clearly, additional tests such as a CT myelogram may be needed to view the spinal cord and spinal nerves. Or a CT myelogram may be ordered for a person who cannot have an MRI because he has a pacemaker or certain implants that rule out the possibility of MRI.

A myelogram is an injection of dye through a lumbar puncture. A specialist injects dye ("contrast") through a small needle into the spinal fluid. The myelographic table may be tilted to move the contrast up and down your spine. The contrast shows up on the x-rays that are taken of your spinal cord and nerves. If your physician or surgeon believes that testing the spinal fluid may be helpful in your diagnosis, then a spinal tap is done as part of the myelogram procedure, and spinal fluid is taken out for testing. A CT scan is usually conducted right after a myelogram, to take advantage of the clear views offered when the contrast dye is in place.

If you are not a patient in the hospital, the myelogram is done as an outpatient procedure, and you will go home afterward. Someone should drive you home after the test.

Some people get what is called a *post-myelogram headache* because a hole has been created in the dura, the covering of the nerves, and spinal fluid continues to leak out after the test. The leakage leads to a pressure drop in the brain, a sagging of the brain, and irritation of the blood vessels and the covering of the brain, which causes a headache. The headache may be avoided and is usually less intense if the patient lies flat for about eight hours rather than standing up or sitting up. The column of fluid is less likely to leak out if the pressure on the hole is decreased, as it is when you lie down.

Today, fortunately, very small needles are used, and the smallest amount of contrast necessary is injected, so headache is less common than it used to be. The headache, when it occurs, may cause nausea and vomiting, dizziness, and a tight feeling behind the eyes. If you get a headache, you should stay in bed another eight to ten hours. The headache usually clears up within twenty-four to forty-eight hours, and if it lasts a long time, it can be treated with a procedure called a *blood patch*, wherein a doctor takes some of the patient's blood and injects the blood in the area where the puncture was made. The blood seals off that area and is quite effective at treating the headache.

Provocative Tests

Chronic back pain is difficult to diagnose because there could be many causes. If the surgeon does not have a good idea of the cause of the patient's pain, then the surgeon doesn't operate because the chance of making the person worse is just as good as the chance of making the patient better. Radiographic imaging tests (X-ray, CT scan, and MRI) are conducted to try to identify specific or isolated radiographic abnormalities (structural abnormalities that show up on the scans). In provocative tests—discogram—the physician will try to re-create or induce the back pain by stimulation of a specific disc to determine whether that particular structure is the source of the pain. The usefulness of predicting success of a surgery in relieving a person's back pain is controversial, and it is not universally accepted by the medical community as a useful test.

Electrodiagnostic Studies

Electrodiagnostic studies can help identify the cause of many problems, including pain, weakness, numbness, and abnormal sensation. Needle electromyographic (EMG) examination and nerve conduction studies are two primary electrodiagnostic tests. The patient does not have to prepare in advance for these tests, although you should tell your physician whether you are taking any blood-thinning medications, have hemophilia, or a cardiac pacemaker.

During an EMG examination, a specialist physician inserts a fine-needle electrode into the muscles to observe the electric activity of the nerve as displayed on a screen and listens to the electric activity over a loudspeaker. The physician can see how well the nerve and the muscle are functioning as a unit. The needles are not used to inject anything, and no electric current runs through them. Insertion of the needles causes some pain, but the test generally does not take long.

In nerve conduction studies, the physician tapes metal electrodes to the skin and then runs a small electric current to the nerve. The physician then observes how the nerve responds to the current. The nerve conduction study looks at how rapidly the signal in the nerve travels from one point to another. It may detect the slowing of the transmission of the signal in particular locations, and that slowing indicates the location of the compressed or irritated nerve.

These studies are used when the nerves are involved, but the doctor is not sure about the cause of the nerve symptoms. They will be helpful in locating the problem. They tend to be used not for back pain, but for nerve symptoms related to the legs or arms. They are useful in identifying nonspinal causes of nerve problems that are not clear with other tests. We use them to rule out peripheral nerve involvement versus more central nerve involvement, to look for nerve compression, say, around the knee or around the hip due to irritation of the nerve root, or for other systemic causes, such as diabetes, as a cause of numbness, weakness, or other systemic conditions.

Nerve conduction studies can be useful for identifying what's wrong with the nerve and where. They can show you, within a few inches, of where the problem is—or they may show just a generalized problem of indeterminate cause.

Nerve conduction studies are useful for testing the upper and lower extremities if someone has pain down the leg (sciatica) and the physician does not know whether the sciatica stems from pressure on a nerve root, some other problem around the spine, pressure on the sciatic nerve around the hip, or pressure on the nerve around the knee. The nerve conduction test will be useful in identifying the problem. If the test showed that pain was coming from pressure on the nerve around the knee, we would treat the nerve around the knee. If it was coming from the nerve around the hip, we would treat the nerve around the hip.

If someone has radiographic evidence of pressure on the nerve root, has diabetes, and the physician is trying to determine whether the nerve root or the diabetes is the problem, then the test can be useful. If the problem is hand numbness, is it carpal tunnel or is the numbness from your hand or from your neck? If it is from carpal tunnel and the hand is numb, we release the nerve at the wrist. Sometimes, nerve conduction studies are not specific and then we have to use our clinical judgment.

Nerve Root Block

Nerve root block, an outpatient procedure, is used to relieve pain. The patient is instructed not to eat or drink anything beginning at midnight the night before the test. Before the test, an IV may be started to provide fluids. In this test, a doctor injects a medication around the nerve root that may be causing pain. The test takes between twenty and thirty minutes.

Discogram

A discogram is a test to irritate a disc to re-create the back pain. The theory is that if stimulation of a specific structure like the disc re-creates the back pain like no other structure around it does, then a fusion or a disc replacement for that particular structure might lead to less back pain. Its limitation is that it can only localize the potential source of somebody's pain—it doesn't predict the outcome of an operation. A discogram will answer the question, "Is this disc causing pain?" It doesn't necessarily tell you that a fusion or disc replacement will relieve the pain.

You should only agree to the discogram if you are willing to have a back operation. The test is conducted to help decide whether you are a candidate for surgery. Therefore, if you are not sure you would be willing to undergo an operation, then you should not have the discogram. It does not make you better; in fact, it is a pain-generating test and a painful test. Neither is it a completely reliable test, in part because pain is subjective, and doctors often can't tell from the patient's response how bad the pain is. Nor is it necessarily reliable in telling us that the disc is the exact spot generating the pain because there are nerves from different locations around several discs. Cross-innervation can make the results of the test confusing, inconsistent, and unreliable in predicting the results of an operation.

Discograms are done one disc at a time because the purpose of the test is to try to locate the cause of the back pain. The patient lies on his or her side on the examining table as the doctor sticks a needle into the center (the nucleus pulposus) of a disc that is to be tested and then injects dye through the needle. The patient is not told beforehand which discs will be tested. The doctor injects and pressurizes the disc to irritate it or to stimulate it. You must determine whether the stimulation causes pain and whether this is the pain that you experience on a regular basis. The doctor asks, "Is this the pain you want to get rid of?" You answer yes or no. Then the needle procedure is repeated on another disc; the doctor asks, "We're going to try it again. Yes or no? Is this the pain? Is this your typical pain? Is this the location?" If it hurts, you say, "Yikes, that hurts, and it is painful, but it is not my pain," or you say, "Yikes, that hurts and is painful, and it could be, might be, my pain," or "Yikes, that hurts and is painful, but I am not sure." So the result at each disc is positive, negative, or indeterminate. A positive response is rare, in which case you would say, "Yes, that's it!" This is a subjective test because you must qualify and quantify your response.

Sometimes x-rays are taken of the discs during the test. In a normal disc, the dye shows the outline of the nucleus pulposus; for an abnormality, such as a rupture or a worn disc, the dye may leak out.

Some doctors perform the discogram on a sedated patient because the test is painful, and they do not want the patient to remember it. The patient is able to participate, but getting a level of sedation that does not alter the patient's abilities to discern or convey their feelings is difficult. Other physicians perform discograms without sedation.

This subjective and painful test carries a slight risk of infection, and the inconsistency in how it is performed, the cross-innervation in the back, and the many other causes of pain in the back raise questions about the test's validity. The degree of useful information obtained from a discogram is controversial. However, if the physician has narrowed down the cause of the pain to a few likely sources and needs one more piece of information to make a decision, then it can be a useful test.

Other Diagnostic Tests

Bone Scan

A bone scan detects bone activity caused by disease, infection, or fracture. For this test, a small amount of radioactive material is injected into a vein in the patient's arm two or three hours before the test begins. When the test begins, the patient lies flat on a table and remains as still as possible. A special camera detects the radioactive material and takes images of the skeletal system. The examination lasts between thirty and sixty minutes.

A bone scan is generally a safe test. A woman who is or who may be pregnant or who is nursing should not have a bone scan unless it is clearly needed.

Facet Blocks

Facet blocks can provide information about where a particular joint is inflamed or irritated. These blocks can also be used to treat pain (and are discussed again in Chapter 6).

You lie on a table for the test. The physician injects local anesthesia into the skin to numb the area and then, guided by x-ray pictures on a monitor, places a needle into the facet joint that your doctor believes may be causing your pain, or near the nerves that travel to that joint. After injecting medication such as lidocaine or steroids through the needle, the physician will ask you about your sensations of discomfort or pain to determine whether the injection has relieved or improved the pain. If it has, then there is a good chance that the pain is coming from that location.

A facet block takes between thirty and sixty minutes. After the test, you can resume your normal activities, but do not take any pain medications for two hours after the procedure so that you can continue to monitor what effect, if any, the procedure has on your pain.

Professionals Who Treat Back Pain

As we said earlier in this chapter, if you are having an acute episode of back pain, your family doctor or internist is the person you should see first. They can handle most of the problems related to the back—probably 90 percent of them. They can prescribe muscle relaxants and pain medications that will help. They can refer you to a physical therapist and order x-rays, and if your pain does not improve, they can refer you to a variety of specialists. Those specialists include physical medicine rehabilitation doctors, called *physiatrists*, who are physicians who specialize in nonoperative treatment of a variety of conditions, including back pain. They can prescribe medications and use a transcutaneous electrical nerve stimulators (TENS) unit for injections and diagnostic and therapeutic blocks and to perform tests such as the EMG / nerve conduction test if that would be indicated. (The TENS device delivers electrical impulses to the body to block the body's pain signals; see Chapter 6.) They can prescribe a physical therapy or medicine program and follow you for that program. Some physiatrists are associated with and work closely with spine surgeons at a spine center and can refer a patient to a surgeon if it is necessary. Physiatrists are specialized in techniques for dealing with back pain.

Neurosurgeons and orthopedic spine surgeons mostly focus on identifying patients with surgically treatable spine conditions. They will often try to reduce your symptoms in the process of trying to decide whether you are a surgical candidate, but they will not ultimately become your primary doctor for back pain. Once they decide that you are not a surgical candidate, they cannot take you on as a permanent patient. The job of a neurosurgeon or an orthopedic surgeon is to identify surgically treatable causes of back and leg pain and then treat them surgically. Most surgeons will be neither qualified in nor interested in the long-term management of nonoperative causes of back pain. They will refer you to other physicians such as a physiatrist and pain treatment specialist or recommend that you continue treatment with your internist.

Referrals, by the way, are done because they are the right thing to do. In some private practices, patients may be referred back and forth. Seldom is there an ulterior motive for a referral, and no money is involved. If your doctor suggests just one specialist and you feel uncomfortable having just one name, then ask for the names of other specialists.

People who are familiar with a community hospital may not be familiar with the differences between a community hospital and a research, academic, and teaching hospital. We are located in a teaching hospital and may be biased, but we will tell you how we see the difference: a research/teaching/academic center has more people and more resources available around the clock. A teaching hospital is up to date on newer technologies, and staff have more experience with the new technologies. Overall, physicians in a teaching hospital have a greater depth and breadth of experience than physicians in community hospitals. People sometimes worry that their care will be compromised in a teaching hospital. But a benefit is that a resident is at the hospital all the time and will be available during the day and night. (By the way, the resident is taught to call his or her superior if there is any doubt.)

The doctor-patient relationship is a professional relationship, but it is based on a lot of the same characteristics as a friendship and in some ways is less and in some ways more complicated than a friendship. There must be a basic level of honest communication between the physician and the patient. You can't get or give good medical care without it. If the patient has a level of communication and trust with the physician, and the physician with the patient, that will allow the physician to care for the patient and will allow the patient to benefit from the physician's care.

The flip side is that there is a level of communication and trust below which the relationship cannot be safe and effective for the provision of health care. In that case, patients may choose not to keep their doctors and doctors may choose not to treat specific patients. If a patient says, "I don't trust you" (and means it), then the physician must reply, "You can't be my patient, and I can't be your doctor." The doctor will recommend qualified doctors for the patient to consider.

Most doctors do their best to offer the multiple dimensions of physical, spiritual, and emotional healing. The bottom line is that you want to know that the doctor has your best interests at heart, will not abandon you, and wants to help you.

Six
Pain Relief and Nonsurgical Treatment

OVER TIME, MOST BACK pain improves on its own. Understandably, people want to be as comfortable as possible while they wait. For people with chronic and recurring back pain, being comfortable involves managing symptoms on an ongoing basis. Studies have shown that activity is one of the best ways to recover from back pain. Anti-inflammatories, muscle relaxants, pain medication, and other drugs can ease the pain. In this chapter, we discuss these medications as well as:

- physical therapy, including aerobic conditioning and muscle strengthening
- posture
- chiropractic treatment
- acupuncture
- massage
- injection procedures
- intradiscal electrothermal therapy
- vertebroplasty/kyphoplasty

We'll also consider the important role of controlling anxiety and stress in treating pain, and we'll discuss how depression can both contribute to back pain and prevent someone from getting better.

Once you have had some episodes of back pain, your first objective ought to be to get through the acute episode. Your second objective is to develop new patterns of behavior to minimize the frequency and disruption of future episodes of pain. Back exercises must be included in your regular routine, and you must make sure that you are correctly performing the activities of daily living such as sitting, standing, and lifting. These essential topics are covered extensively in Chapter 7. Exercising and paying attention to ergonomics usually translates into less frequent symptoms that last less time. You also need to develop a strategy and plan to deal with any future episodes of back pain. A strategy might include an anti-inflammatory medication, short-term rest, heat—whatever you find to be most effective.

Some pain comes as a surprise, while other pain can be anticipated. If you know that a specific activity will cause back pain, then that pain is anticipated. If you also know that certain types of medications or treatments are useful in eliminating or reducing the back pain that results from this activity, you might want to start the medication before you do that activity or soak in a hot tub after you have done that activity to avoid the pain. If you have a lot of back pain every time you rake leaves, for example, and you have found that an anti-inflammatory medication reduces pain after you have the back pain, you might want to take the medication *before* you rake, so you have a minimum of pain while you rake and afterward. Continue to take the medication on schedule for some period after the activity, as well.

Some episodes of pain are the result of new activities or extremes of activity. You have to be smart and think about what things you can do and how you can modify the way you do them. In addition, what kinds of things can you *not* do? You will need to find substitutes for them or find an adaptive way to do those things. You might take anti-inflammatory medications before a new activity (such as helping your daughter move into her college dormitory). In addition, if you are lifting and moving boxes, you need to use proper lifting techniques and you may need to use assistive devices such as a dolly to avoid stressing your back. If you are shoveling snow, raking leaves, or pulling weeds for the first time this year, and you are not in shape, you are asking your body to do something that it is not prepared to do and to do it for a long time. Back pain in those circumstances is normal; however, by taking measures beforehand to avoid pain, and by doing these tasks in a slightly different way, long-term consequences can be avoided.

For chronic pain, anti-inflammatory medications and back exercises are helpful in keeping people comfortable. Some chronic back pain only responds to consistent treatment, such as exercising the back each day (see Chapter 7).

As your back strengthens and your back pain lessens, as you can do things like physical therapy and back exercises, as the inflammation goes down, you can gradually do activities without pain, and your ability to perform more strenuous activities will steadily increase. Early on in the recovery process, you will hit and go beyond the limits of your physical capabilities and have recurrence of pain. The more you work on it, however, your endurance will increase, the less pain you will have, and the more active you can be.

Medications

Nonsteroidal anti-inflammatory medications (NSAIDs) such as ibuprofen, Motrin, and Aleve are often the place to begin when treating pain. For people with stomach problems, Tylenol (acetaminophen) is a reasonable alternative, although it does not relieve inflammation.

The NSAIDs have two mechanisms of action. (1) They block your brain's perception of pain. (2) They reduce inflammation at the affected area—the sprained or inflamed joints, muscles, or tendons. Because they have two mechanisms of action, they are often more effective than Tylenol, which blocks pain but does not reduce inflammation. It takes between ten and fourteen days for the anti-inflammatory mechanism to have its full effect through reduction of inflammation through constant use. To get the full benefit of the pain-relieving properties of NSAIDs, this cumulative effect must be permitted to occur. That's why it's important to take the medication regularly for the recommended period.

As long as you are not having side effects from the medication, continue to take it for at least two to three weeks, even if it does not seem to be working the way you would like it to work. In two to three weeks, you will be able to tell what additive effect the medication has had on your inflammation. Many people give up on it after a day or two, thinking that it is not working, when in fact the effect that the physician is looking for isn't going to kick in or be apparent for at least two weeks. The prescribed dosages of NSAIDs are higher than over-the-counter dosages to give the maximum effect of the medication and to allow a more even distribution of anti-inflammatory effects of the drug over time.

Tylenol blocks the perception of pain; it has no cumulative effect. This applies to narcotics as well, which only work over the course of the single dose; they do not have an additive effect over time. Narcotics also have undesirable side effects, such as constipation, lethargy, and depression, which may discourage you from moving around. Because moving around is ultimately the best thing you can do for your back, these are highly undesirable side effects.

Anti-inflammatory medications may cause easy bleeding or bruising because they affect blood platelets. They can also cause gastric upset, heartburn, and ulcers. If taken in high dosages or for a long time they may affect liver and kidney function. People taking NSAIDs should ask their doctor how often and when to have their liver and kidney function checked. NSAIDs affect the heart and may have an effect on blood pressure, so people who have had heart failure or have marginal heart failure need to check with their doctor or cardiologist about heart function and whether it is a good idea to take an NSAID. Most of the side effects are uncommon and the majority of people can take anti-inflammatory medications at a prescription dose for long periods of time without any problems.

Not every anti-inflammatory medication works for everyone. A doctor will try to find the best fit for a particular person. The doctor looks for minimal side effects with maximum therapeutic benefits and maximum pain relief. If one anti-inflammatory isn't working, either because of intolerable side effects or because it is not reducing pain, your doctor may prescribe another one. Some people who do not have any significant pain relief with one anti-inflammatory will have dramatic relief with another. And a portion of people who have significant side effects with one will have minimal side effects with another.

Muscle relaxants are another category of medication. They reduce muscle spasm and allow patients to be more mobile, but they do not address the cause of the pain. Many have side effects or cause drowsiness or inability to function normally, but they do reduce muscle spasms in the back. If a muscle relaxant causes drowsiness if taken during the day, then take the medication at night to help with sleep. Newer muscle relaxants have less of a sedating effect, so they are probably more useful during the day. Heating pads, shower massage, and other local treatments, such as hot baths or whirlpools, can also help with back spasms. Again, they do not address the inflammation or the root source of the pain, but they can be a useful addition to some other medications and forms of treatment. These methods should only be used if they make you feel better.

Physical Therapy

This section on physical therapy is short because Chapter 7 is devoted to this medical specialty. Major benefits can be gained from physical therapy, and many doctors prescribe physical therapy for treating back pain and functional problems. Physical therapy should be goal oriented and limited in time, which means we prefer patients spend their time returning to a normal level of activity rather than traveling to a physical therapy office. And proper physical therapy accomplishes exactly that (see Chapter 7).

Chiropractic Treatment, Acupuncture, and Other Complementary Medicines

Western medicine has not yet produced much useful data about the benefits of chiropractic treatment, acupuncture, and similar modalities. Yet, many of our patients see a chiropractor, especially if they have not found pain relief through the usual routes. Most chiropractors we know will not only do manipulations or massages

Back Pain at a Glance: What Kind of Exercises Help to Prevent and Relieve Back Pain?

With any kind of exercise, it is essential to start slowly and to allow the muscles to warm up and loosen before increasing the pace or load.

- General aerobic activity such as walking and swimming helps keeps the heart and lungs healthy and generally helps you stay in shape.
- Exercises designed to strengthen and maintain tone in back muscles and the abdomen help to prevent injury and pain.
- Pilates focuses on strengthening abdominal muscles and back muscles, providing core strength and flexibility.
- Yoga increases flexibility.
- The McKenzie method of passive end-range stretching exercises are designed to strengthen the back muscles.
- Exercising using the Swedish ball strengthens the abs and improves balance and overall coordination.

but also provide instruction in back exercises. A chiropractor's treatment is often similar to a physical therapist's, although chiropractors emphasize manipulations. We're not sure whether chiropractic has any benefits over standard physical therapy in treating a lower back, but we know that in most instances it is not harmful and can be a reasonable part of a broader program to return to health. It should not be used to the exclusion of other treatments such as medications, physical therapy, and exercise.

Acupuncture is a Chinese regimen that has been effective for centuries in reducing pain and inducing anesthesia for certain procedures. Within the scientific community, there is some skepticism about acupuncture's effectiveness because there is little evidence one way or the other that compares it with more traditional Western techniques. There is at present a large amount of research into acupuncture's effectiveness or ineffectiveness.

The benefit of any approach that reduces pain, ultimately, is activity. To recover well, you want an active, not a passive, rehabilitation program. All of your efforts should be directed toward resuming a *normal level of activity*. A short-term approach to reduce pain may make you less active. Narcotics may help relieve pain but sedate you or make you lethargic. Muscle relaxants may help relax your muscles, but they may make you tired. In the long term, these counterproductive approaches prevent you from getting back to normal. This also applies to passive modalities such as acupuncture or manipulation, heating pads, or electrical stimulation or massage. Mostly, you feel better while you are having these procedures done, but ultimately, they do not increase your level of activity. You may feel better for five or ten minutes, but later on you don't feel any better, and you won't be able to be more active.

Injection Procedures

Epidural injections are sometimes used to treat back pain. They are most useful for leg pain such as radicular pain or sciatica, and they are not as useful for back pain. (Radicular pain radiates along the nerve and is often due to inflammation or other irritation of the nerve root.) Steroids are injected in the epidural space in the spinal canal near the nerves.

When the facet joint is the source of pain, we can use facet blocks as a temporary or permanent attempt to relieve pain (see also Chapter 5). The doctor can inject lidocaine or steroids around the facet joint and see whether pain is reduced. Lidocaine usually numbs it up completely, but only temporarily, whereas steroids are injected to try to reduce the inflammation around the joint permanently.

The facet joints have cross-enervation, so it is not always possible to isolate the source of the pain if several of the joints look arthritic on imaging tests. If the facet block works temporarily, however, the doctor may feel more confident about the source of the pain and may do an ablation, which involves burning the nerve endings around the joint. Ablations are done with a high-temperature probe like a cautery that heats up nerve endings around the joint and kills them. Ablations in some instances are an alternative to a major operation with a long recovery. If the ablation doesn't help, the operation can still be done and the operation is no more difficult than it would have been.

It can be difficult to isolate the problematic structure. Another problem is that a single structure may not be causing the problem. When someone has arthritis at multiple levels, several structures are involved. Older people tend to have multiple levels of involvement, which decreases the chance of success from an injection procedure, whereas in younger people, the facet block can be effective, especially if the pain is brought on by activities or an injury.

Intradiscal Electrothermal Therapy

Intradiscal electrothermal therapy (IDET) uses a wire called an electrothermal catheter to deliver heat directly to a disc. There have been no adequate studies of the outcomes of this procedure; therefore, we do not recommend it at this time.

Vertebroplasty and Kyphoplasty

Vertebral compression fractures from osteoporosis and myeloma are sometimes treated with a vertebroplasty or kyphoplasty procedure. Studies report that these procedures are successful in reducing pain and improving quality of life. In both procedures, bone cement, about the consistency of toothpaste, is injected into the vertebral body; then, over several minutes, the cement hardens and stabilizes the bone. A physician must take a number of considerations into account when recommending one procedure or the other. If a patient has a bone fragment in the spinal canal, compression of the spinal cord, or severe deformity of the spinal column because of collapsed vertebrae, neither kyphoplasty nor vertebroplasty can be performed.

In vertebroplasty, the surgeon uses x-ray guidance to inject cement directly into the cracked or broken vertebral through a hollow instrument into the patient's back. The cement fills the cracked parts of the bone and essentially stabilizes it when it becomes hardened. This procedure does not restore the height of the vertebral body to its original size, so the person remains shortened, and if there is any bend (angulation) at that level, it is not corrected.

Kyphoplasty is a more complicated and technically demanding procedure. Using x-ray guidance, the surgeon places a hollow instrument in the vertebral body and then inserts a deflated balloon through the needle into the vertebra. Once the balloon is in place, it is inflated, in the hope that it will expand and lift the collapsed vertebra, possibly restoring some of the height of the vertebral body. In this process, a space is created in the vertebra, which acts as a container for the cement. After the balloon is deflated and taken out, the surgeon fills that space with cement. Thus, rather than filling up only the cracks and canals in the bone, as with vertebroplasty, in kyphoplasty the surgeon is also filling the space created by the balloon.

Another difference between vertebroplasty and kyphoplasty is that during the vertebroplasty procedure the cement is injected under very high pressure. The surgeon must push the cement through a small needle into a limited space in the vertebral body using an enormous amount of pressure, whereas with a kyphoplasty, the surgeon places a balloon in the vertebra and creates a space—a hole—before injecting the cement, so the procedure does not require the application of high pressure. If there is any question about the integrity of bone on the side of the spinal canal, kyphoplasty is the safer procedure, and it also has the advantage of potentially restoring the height of the vertebral body.

Psychological Factors

Stress and tension magnify back pain, and anything that leads to less tension and less stress helps to relieve back pain. Relaxation therapy, such as massages and acupuncture, reduces tension and stress. Soaking in a bath, taking a leisurely walk, talking with a friend, reading a good book—all of the things we have learned to do to reduce the normal stress of daily life can come to our aid if we are in pain because our muscles are tight with stress.

As we have seen, for most people, back pain lasts about three months, gradually improving over time. Some people, however, have continued back pain for over six months, and for many of them, the pain does not get better. This small group of people uses the majority of medical, financial, and societal resources for back pain.

Some people are more likely to have continued pain despite treatments that, in most instances, would lead to relief of pain and resumption of normal activities. Someone who is unhappy with his or her life may not respond to standard treatment for back pain.

Some people have "fear avoidance," an exaggerated fear of pain, and they even avoid treatment that would benefit them in the long run, such as physical therapy or gradually resuming normal activities. Some people are psychologically distressed or depressed. Addressing underlying psychological conditions such as depression and anxiety will improve or resolve their back pain.

Everything is more difficult for people who are miserable in their jobs. Finally, if there are legal claims or workers' compensation, and the person will benefit from not getting better, or if there is some financial or psychosocial advantage to being disabled, the person is less likely to get better.

People in any of these unhappy situations can be difficult for doctors to identify, but it is important that these issues are recognized and the individual is referred for treatment for their psychosocial problem as part of their treatment for ongoing back problems. Often a psychosocial problem is the primary disease in need of treatment. If we do not address or treat that problem, especially if the problem is psychological, then the person will not get better. If we treat that problem with medications and psychological counseling, their back symptoms have a better chance of improving. These people are either manifesting a primary psychological disease through another symptom (such as back pain), or their psychological issues are severe enough to prevent them from having a normal recovery from disease, just like it is preventing them from functioning normally in their lives. We need to help them cope not only with their back but also with other aspects of life.

Seven
Physical Therapy for Pain, Strength, and Function

Kristin R. Archer, Ph.D., D.P.T.

WHEN CARING FOR PEOPLE with acute or chronic and recurring back pain, doctors often prescribe physical therapy (sometimes called PT) as part of treatment. Physical therapy also is commonly prescribed to help people recover from back surgery. In this chapter, we discuss both of these uses of PT.

Physical therapy is a rehabilitation specialty provided by licensed health care professionals. Therapists may hold a bachelor's degree, master's degree (MSPT), or doctorate degree in physical therapy (DPT), and many have additional certification as an orthopedic specialist (OCS). Health insurance generally covers much of the cost of physical therapy.

Physical therapists assess and treat various back conditions. If a physical therapist is treating your back problem, you can count on the therapist to provide guidance, support, and education to help you:

- move better (mobility)
- move more safely
- reduce pain and discomfort

- function better
- avoid disability

The American Physical Therapy Association (APTA) states that physical therapy includes:

- Examining individuals with impairment, functional limitation, disability, or other health-related conditions to determine a diagnosis, prognosis, and intervention.
- Alleviating impairment and functional limitation by designing, implementing, and modifying therapeutic interventions.
- Preventing injury, impairment, functional limitation, and disability, and promoting and maintaining fitness, health, and quality of life in people of all ages.
- Engaging in consultation, education, and research.

Meet the Physical Therapist

What can you expect on your first visit to a physical therapist? First, the therapist will take a thorough medical history. Usually, the physical therapist and your doctor will communicate with each other before your visit to the therapist, and the therapist will know about the diagnostic tests or surgical procedures that have been performed on you. If not, the therapist will contact your physician during or after your initial visit. You can bring radiology reports and other relevant information (such as test results and use of medications) with you to share with your therapist.

After taking a medical history, the therapist will perform a careful evaluation of your spine. The evaluation will include an assessment of posture and body mechanics, muscle strength, range of motion (often called "R-O-M," this is an indication of how far you are able to move or stretch), nerve function, and ability to perform the activities of daily living.

The physical therapist will also ask questions about your pain. Specifically, a therapist will want to know the frequency and severity of your pain, what makes your pain better and worse throughout the day, and if you have any radiating leg or arm pain or numbness and tingling. The therapist may ask you to rate your daily pain on a scale from 0 to 10, with 0 being no pain and 10 being pain so severe you would need to go to the hospital. Keeping track of your pain and sharing information about the frequency, intensity, and aggravators of pain with your therapist is essential. This information will help your therapist not only understand your condition but also choose the most effective interventions to treat your pain and functional limitations (sometimes called *disability*).

Don't be surprised if you feel an increased level of pain or discomfort after the evaluation. Sometimes the movement and positions of the initial visit aggravate symptoms. Tell your therapist about any increase in symptoms. He or she can use modalities (methods or approaches to treatment) such as thermotherapy (heat application) and cryotherapy (cold application) to help alleviate your discomfort. After the initial evaluation, go home and rest for the remainder of the day and take any medication recommended by your doctor.

After evaluating you, the therapist will explain his or her findings and discuss the appropriate treatment options. The duration and frequency of physical therapy treatment can vary from only three or four visits devoted to teaching you exercises and proper lifting techniques, to additional visits in which modalities such as ultrasound and massage are used to reduce your discomfort. The major benefit of physical therapy comes from learning the exercise program and then doing the exercises on your own at home. Physical therapy sessions can be expensive and time consuming, so therapists rely on their patients to faithfully do their prescribed exercises and follow other instructions to avoid injury, decrease pain, and improve function.

Choosing a therapist that you trust and feel safe with is important. Therapists have different perspectives and educational backgrounds, and treatment is different depending on which therapist you see. Your physician will probably recommend one or more physical therapy groups or a specific therapist, but you can also collect word-of-mouth recommendations from people you trust. Ultimately, you are in charge of your rehabilitation. An important part of being an active participant is feeling comfortable with the physical therapist you choose.

Physical Therapy Interventions for Daily Living

A study of Los Angeles County firefighters emphasized the importance of exercise for a healthy back. The firefighters were divided into two groups. One group was physically active and did back exercises, and one group was not active and did not do back exercises. The inactive group had back problems more frequently, and their symptoms lasted longer than the firefighters who regularly did back exercises.

Most people with back pain are out of shape and need a back exercise program. Physical therapists focus on active modalities such as back exercises, and they teach techniques that will help you maintain a healthy back. If your pain is due to improper lifting, sitting, twisting, or other activities, then becoming more active and learning the proper lifting techniques and ergonomics (how to sit, stand, and move) allow you to protect your back and prevent a recurrence. An important part of getting back to normal is learning the back exercise program, learning the proper lifting techniques, and learning how to sleep and sit properly to protect your back— and then integrating these elements into your daily routine.

Back Pain at a Glance: What's the Best Way to Perform Back Exercises?

- Do the exercise on a firm surface covered with a thin mat (such as a yoga mat) or a heavy blanket.
- Put a pillow under your neck if that makes you more comfortable.
- Only do exercises that are recommended by your doctor or physical therapist.
- Allow muscles to loosen up and warm up: begin slowly and do the exercises in the recommended order. Heat treatments before exercise help warm up muscles. (Cold muscles are more prone to injury.)
- Don't overdo it, especially in the beginning. Start slowly and carefully, and do only a few repetitions.
- The exercises may cause slight discomfort, lasting a couple of minutes. This is expected and acceptable, especially when you are first starting out.
- If the pain is severe, or if it lasts more than a couple of minutes, stop the exercises and check with your doctor.

Back Exercise Program

A back exercise program includes three components: (1) flexibility (stretching), (2) strength (the ability to exert force), and (3) endurance (the ability to perform activities repeatedly without fatigue or pain). Your physical therapist will tell you which exercises are right for you, how often to exercise, and how many times to repeat each exercise (called *repetitions*). Different exercises are recommended, depending on your spine condition, the type of pain you have, and whether your pain is acute or chronic. General aerobic conditioning, back and abdominal muscle strengthening, and back and hip stretching exercises are all useful.

Proper Lifting Techniques

A physical therapist will evaluate your lifting technique on either the first or the second visit. The best way to lift an object is as follows:

- Stand close to the object, with feet firmly planted, and in a wide stance.
- Bend your knees and keep your back straight.
- Make sure you have a secure grip on the object and keep the object as close to you as possible.
- Lift the object by slowly straightening your knees. Avoid jerking your body.
- When standing upright, shift your feet to turn instead of twisting.

This technique can be difficult to follow when lifting objects from the trunk of your car, so, when lifting items in and out of your trunk, take the following steps:

- Place your foot on the bumper of your car for support if the bumper is not too high.
- Store items in the trunk close to the bumper.
- Lift items onto the car frame first and then lift them from the car frame to your arms.

- If you must reach something located deep inside the trunk, brace yourself on the car with one arm while reaching.

Proper body mechanics when pushing or pulling objects is equally important. When pushing an object, bend your knees so your arms are level with the object. Maintain a straight spine and walk forward pushing the object in front of you using your legs. When pulling an object, bend your knees so your arms are level with the object. Maintain a straight spine and walk *backward*, pulling the object with your body weight rather than with your arms or your back. Whenever you can, push rather than pull—and remember to pace yourself and take frequent breaks.

Proper Sleeping Positions

A physical therapist will help you find the best sleeping position to reduce your pain. Most people find the benefit from these two positions: Sleep on your back with your knees bent and a pillow under your knees, or sleep on your side with your knees bent and a pillow between your legs. Both positions decrease the pressure on the spinal discs and lower back.

If side sleeping provides the most benefit, then make sure your legs rest on top of each other with your knees bent or have your top leg slightly forward. Avoid resting your top knee on the bed and sleeping with your arms under your neck and head. A pillow placed behind the body and tucked under the back and hips can help to keep you from rolling out of position. When sleeping on your back, avoid sleeping with your arms over your head, because this position puts too much stress on your shoulders and neck. Sleeping on your stomach is not recommended. If you are lying on your stomach for a short time, place a pillow under your lower abdominal muscles to help reduce pressure on the spine.

Changing positions in bed can be difficult for people with back pain. To reduce discomfort, always use the *log roll* when turning: Keep your back straight and avoid twisting when rolling from side to side and onto your back. For example, if you are lying on your left side, bend your knees and log roll onto your back, keeping your spine straight and your shoulders in line with your hips. Then, with your knees bent, log roll onto your right side. The log roll can also be used for getting in and out of bed. If getting out of bed on the right side, log roll onto your right side, and use your left hand to push yourself up onto your right elbow. Slowly drop your lower legs off the bed as you push yourself up onto your right hand and into a sitting position. Scoot to the edge of the bed and place both feet on the floor. Use your legs, and not your back, to come to a standing position.

When returning to bed, move backward until the back of your legs are touching the bed. Bend slowly at the knees and hips, not at the back, and lower yourself onto the bed. Then, slowly swing your lower legs onto the bed at the same time that you descend onto your elbow and then into a side-lying position. From a side-lying position, you can log roll onto your back or onto your other side.

Proper Sitting Techniques

Sitting places stress and pressure on the ligaments and discs of the lower back. Over time, this stress can cause them to stretch and weaken, and they will no longer be able to protect your back. To help minimize this stress and avoid injury, you need to maintain your normal spinal curves when sitting. As described in Chapter 1, these normal curves are at your neck, midback, and lower back.

Slouching or sliding down in your chair places strain on your back. To avoid slouching, keep your ears, shoulders, and hips aligned. Make sure you have a proper chair that fits you and try to choose a chair that provides support for your lower back. If lumbar support is not available, place a lumbar roll or a rolled towel in the small of your back. Some people find a seat wedge useful. This is a triangular wedge to sit on with the widest part placed at the back of the chair. The wedge tilts the pelvis to maintain the proper position of the lower back.

In choosing a chair, find one that allows your feet to be flat on the floor with your knees at the same level as your hips. Ideally, your hips and knees should be at a 90-degree angle, and weight should be evenly distributed on both hips. Avoid sitting in soft chairs and on couches where your hips drop below your knees. If a chair is too high for you, place your feet on a small stool or box to help maintain correct sitting posture. Remember to take objects out of your back pockets (don't sit on them) and avoid crossing your legs and sitting on your legs. Take frequent breaks by standing up and stretching. Placing your hands on the small of your back and arching backward can sometimes help reduce stiffness. Make sure your legs don't get cold while you are sitting, because they can cramp and become tense.

When working at a desk, use a chair that swivels or turns. This is a much better option than twisting your body to reach objects. If you need to turn, try moving your body as a single unit. Keep your hips and feet pointed in the same direction when you are moving.

Computer keyboards should be placed directly in front of you. Items should always be placed within easy sight and access, and heavy books should be arranged close by and not on a shelf above your head.

If you are often on the telephone, you may want to consider using a headset or headphones. If you constantly twist to answer your telephone, you can reduce the stress on your lower back by moving the phone so it is positioned in front of you. When you are on the phone, do not use your head to hold the receiver. Support the arm that is holding the phone by placing that elbow on the desk or armrest; keep your neck in good alignment.

Getting in and out of a chair can be difficult for people with back pain. To get out of a chair, slide to the edge of the chair. With your chin slightly tucked in and one foot placed in front of the other, straighten your hips and knees to lift yourself from the chair. If the chair has armrests, use your hands to assist you, and remember to keep your back straight. Avoid bending at the back or leaning too far forward. Think about reaching the top of your head straight up toward the ceiling. To return to a sitting position, move backward until the backs of your legs are touching the chair. Place one foot in front of the other; reach back with your hands and, keeping your back straight, lower yourself to the edge of the chair by bending at the hips and knees. Then slide back into the chair.

Physical Therapy Interventions for Pain Relief

Mobilization, Hot and Cold Therapy, and TENS Therapy

In addition to teaching back exercise programs and proper lifting, sleeping, and sitting techniques, physical therapists often use therapeutic interventions to reduce pain and disability. These interventions include joint and soft tissue mobilization (manual or hands-on therapy) and modalities such as hot and cold packs, ultrasound, and TENS units ("TENS" stands for transcutaneous electrical nerve stimulators).

Mobilization (both joint and soft tissue) is a hands-on treatment performed with the patient resting in a comfortable position. Therapists use their hands to locate the area of dysfunction and then apply pressure with their hands in the appropriate direction. Techniques are performed at a slow speed, and the patient can ask the therapist to stop the movement if he or she experiences any discomfort. After mobilization, stretching and strengthening exercises are done to maintain joint range of motion and prevent and relieve pain. Mobilization is safe to perform on most painful and restricted joints and soft tissue; to be safe, the therapist will perform an assessment before mobilization begins.

Joint mobilization is a manual technique used by a physical therapist to treat joint dysfunction such as stiffness or pain. A therapist applies passive movement to a joint through gentle oscillations or distraction, gliding, or a sustained stretch. Mobilization is used to release tension and stiffness, decrease pain, and increase the mobility (that is, movability) of a joint. *Soft tissue mobilization* is a manual technique used by a therapist to treat soft tissue dysfunction such as pain or reduced tissue mobility. A therapist applies pressure to soft tissue (muscles, tendons, or ligaments) through various movements of the hand and fingers such as gliding, kneading, deep friction, percussion, rolling, or sustained stretching. Mobilization is used to restore tissue strength and mobility, decrease tension and spasm, increase blood flow, reduce adhesions and scar tissue, and reduce pain and discomfort.

The goal of *therapeutic modalities* is to provide an optimal environment for healing and injury repair. These modalities complement mobilization techniques and back exercises. A therapist performs an evaluation to find out which modality is likely to be helpful and then applies or supervises the application of the modality. Common modalities are superficial and deep thermotherapy (heat application) and cryotherapy (cold application). Superficial heat can be provided using moist hot packs, whirlpool, and paraffin (warm wax). Superficial heating agents elevate the skin and tissue temperature within 1 or 2 cm of the skin surface. These agents are usually applied for fifteen to twenty minutes. Ultrasound is a method for providing deep heat. Ultrasound uses sound waves to produce heat in deep tissue, to depths of 3 cm or more, and is usually applied for between five and fifteen minutes. Heat is applied to promote healing, decrease pain, and relax muscles through increased blood flow. It is commonly used for people who have pain lasting from six to twelve weeks, chronic inflammatory conditions (lasting longer than twelve weeks), muscle spasms or guarding (rigidity), or decreased range of motion.

Cryotherapy, or cold application, is usually applied for five to thirty minutes. Cryotherapy cools both superficial and deep tissues. Ice packs, ice massage, ice immersion, controlled cold compression units, and whirlpool are all used to accomplish cooling. Cold agents can penetrate tissue to depths up to 5 cm, depending on which agent is used and how long it is in place. Cold methods produce the following four sensations in this order: cold, burning, aching, and numbness. The purpose of cryotherapy is to reduce pain and inflammation, decrease muscle spasms, and reduce spasticity through decreased blood flow. Cryotherapy is recommended for acute injuries and is usually applied during the first twenty-four to seventy-two hours after an injury. Cold application may also be used to treat muscle spasms or guarding, spasticity, and edema (swelling).

TENS units produce electrical stimulation to decrease pain, increase blood flow, and promote healing. Most units are battery powered and are small enough to be worn. Patches of electrodes are placed over the back or other involved areas and an electrical current runs through the electrodes to try to block the nerve pain fibers—to overwhelm them so they can stop firing. Patients may experience a range of sensations that include mild to strong tingling, burning, or even muscle contraction.

TENS and other modalities may make you feel good while you are having them done, but they have not been proven to have any long-lasting effect or to alter the natural history of back pain. If they help, it's fine to use them. But if it doesn't feel good, it shouldn't be done.   .

McKenzie, Pilates, Swiss Ball, and Aquatic Therapy

In physical therapy, you might encounter such therapies as the McKenzie method, Pilates, Swiss ball therapy, and aquatic therapy. The McKenzie method starts with an evaluation that can "classify" most patients' back conditions by the level of pain or limitation that results from repeated movements, positions, and activities. Patients are classified as having a postural, dysfunction, or derangement syndrome.

A postural syndrome is characterized by pain that results from prolonged postures or positions, such as slouching, while range of motion is usually full and pain free. Repeated movements do not change symptoms in people with postural syndrome, and pain relief is usually immediate with therapy. A dysfunction syndrome is characterized by pain and loss of motion only at the very end range of movement, such as at the end of lumbar flexion (bending forward) or lumbar extension (bending backward). When the person moves away from the end range, pain usually decreases. The derangement classification occurs when a person's pain is constant and increases and decreases with certain movements. For example, if a person has a posterior derangement, pain will increase or radiate out from the back and down into the hips and legs as the person bends forward and decrease or centralize (just in the back) when he or she bends backward.

The McKenzie treatment for each syndrome includes a series of individualized exercises. Active patient involvement is emphasized, which limits the number of visits to the clinic. Ultimately, most patients learn how to treat themselves by gaining hands-on knowledge about minimizing the risk of recurrence and rapidly dealing with recurrence if it occurs.

Pilates is an exercise method based on the work of Joseph Pilates, a German-American who developed his exercise method in the twentieth century. The Pilates method uses spring-based machines and floor exercises. Pilates involves concentrating, coordinating breath and movement, and using the mind to control the muscles of the body. The exercises are designed to increase flexibility and endurance, strengthen muscles, and improve posture. Pilates exercises are particularly useful in teaching people to be aware of their breath and the alignment of their spine and in helping them to strengthen the deep abdominal and back muscles. Keeping these muscles strong is helpful in alleviating and preventing back pain. Pilates programs usually involve an ordered series of exercises that work the entire body and are designed to have minimal impact on the joints.

Since the Pilates method was not originally intended for people with back pain, we recommend starting a Pilates program under the supervision of a physical therapist. Therapists can become trained in Pilates through various methods, ranging from a simple weekend course to one- to three-year certification programs. Experience and training count here. Do not hesitate to ask your therapist how they were trained in Pilates or about his or her qualifications as a Pilates practitioner.

Swiss ball therapy (also called physio ball, gymnic ball, or stability ball) uses an exercise ball to help strengthen and develop the core body muscles that stabilize the spine. Swiss balls are inflatable and are made of vinyl or plastic. The size of the ball varies depending on a person's height and weight and type of exercise program being performed. Usually the size is chosen based on a person's sitting position on the ball, where hips and knees are at or slightly greater than a 90-degree angle (thighs are parallel to the ground or pointing down slightly), with feet flat on the floor. The exercise ball introduces an element of instability into certain exercises; overcoming this instability over time strengthens the muscles used to stay balanced on the Swiss ball.

The exercise ball also enhances a person's awareness of the relative position of different parts of the body (this sense is called *proprioception*). Improved proprioception in turn improves balance and increases a person's confidence in moving through their environment safely and without pain. The benefits of Swiss ball exercise for people with low back pain include:

- a simple and versatile way to start moving again after an episode of back pain
- improved muscle strength
- greater flexibility and range of motion of the spine
- enhanced balance and coordination of core muscle groups used to stabilize the spine and control proper posture while using the exercise ball
- increased tendency to maintain a neutral spine position during exercise

Aquatic therapy or pool therapy can be used to complement a traditional physical therapy program. Exercises are performed in a heated pool where the buoyancy of the water supports the weight of the body and takes the load off the joints and spine. *Unloading* minimizes the weight placed on the spine, which decreases pain and reduces the risk of injury from unintentional movements during exercise. The water provides resistance, so aquatic exercises can help increase strength and endurance or help a person maintain conditioning during recovery from an injury. People who have acute or chronic back pain often need to go into the water for exercise because water allows them to be more active than they can be outside of the water. Aquatic programs consist of various stretching, strengthening, and mobility exercises.

Physical Therapy for Acute Pain

If your back pain is not relieved by rest, anti-inflammatory medications, and a gradual return to normal activities, your physician may refer you to a physical therapist. Early in treatment, physical therapists often focus on pain relief by using mobilization techniques (joint and soft tissue), massage, gentle exercises, and therapeutic modalities. Modalities such as hot packs, ultrasound, or TENS may be applied to the lower back at the start of the treatment session. Ice packs or ice massage may also be used at the end of a session to relieve any pain or stiffness from the therapy session. Therapists usually provide education on proper lifting, sitting, sleeping, and posture to reduce pain and disability.

Physical therapists will then focus on an exercise program that combines trunk stabilization, trunk strengthening, and aerobic conditioning. The goal is to learn a comprehensive home exercise program so you can return to full activity. How to *abdominal brace* is one of the first exercises a physical therapist will demonstrate. Abdominal bracing, or hollowing, uses intra-abdominal pressure to provide stability and protection to the lumbar spine during movement. While you lie on your back, side, or stomach, you will be instructed to tighten the muscles in your lower abdomen and buttocks. You may be asked to tilt your pelvis backward slightly, to flatten your back. This movement should never cause discomfort or increase pain. The purpose of the bracing and slight pelvic movement is to control and maintain a neutral spine position or normal low back curve while breathing. Bracing, or hollowing, is usually held for five to ten seconds in the early stages and gradually increased to sixty seconds as the person begins to master the technique. A physical therapist will tell you how many repetitions to do for bracing, and how many times a day to do it.

Once you master abdominal bracing, or hollowing, you will generally progress to moving your arms and legs to increase muscular endurance. A common progression includes abdominal bracing with single- and double-arm elevation, single- and double-heel slides, single- and double-knee raises, cross-arm knee pushing, and alternating arm raises and leg kicks. Bracing can also be performed lying on the stomach with a pillow under the lower abdomen, lying on the side, or up in a quadruped position (on hands and knees). In quadruped, progression after bracing can include moving the body forward and backward as far as possible, reaching one arm out in front of the body, reaching one leg out behind the body, and eventually reaching with the opposite arm and leg. If for some reason lying on the floor or being in the quadruped position is uncomfortable or painful, bracing can be learned in a more functional position, such as sitting or standing.

Depending on the length of time in physical therapy and a person's pain level, trunk and hip strengthening exercises may be incorporated into a treatment program. The most common strengthening exercises include various forms of abdominal curl-ups or sit-ups, bridging exercises (lifting the hips from the floor after bracing), and exercises lying on the stomach that focus on the spine extensors and hip muscles. These exercises on the stomach often start with gluteal sets (tightening the buttock muscles and holding the contraction for a specified number of seconds) and progress to a single arm or leg lift, an opposite arm and leg lift, both arm or leg lifting, and an upper body lift. Some patients may even progress to the superman exercise, where both arms and both legs are lifted off the ground.

In addition to a comprehensive stabilization and strengthening program, people with acute back pain will be encouraged by therapists to participate in an aerobic exercise program. Such a program usually involves walking, riding a bicycle, or water aerobics. The goal is to gradually increase the amount and intensity of pain-free aerobic conditioning so people can return to their normal level of activity. A program may also include flexibility exercises, especially stretching exercises focusing on the hip flexors (front part of the leg) and extensors (back part of the leg). These can be performed in various positions, such as standing, sitting, kneeling, or lying on the back or stomach.

Every person will have an exercise program tailored to his or her specific needs. *Consult a physician before beginning any new exercise program and only do exercises recommended by your doctor or physical therapist.* An essential component of an exercise program is performing the exercises at home as prescribed. It is also important to keep up with your exercises even after your pain subsides. Maintaining stability, strength, and flexibility is essential for both avoiding chronic pain and not re-injuring your back in the future.

Physical Therapy for Chronic Pain

Chronic lower back pain is characterized as pain lasting longer than three months. Chronic pain is different from acute pain because people with chronic pain often experience some type of emotional distress, even anxiety or depression. Chronic lower back pain can be difficult to treat and is often the reason people seek care from physicians, surgeons, and physical therapists. A main contributor to chronic pain is physical deconditioning (weakness). That is why physical therapy for people with chronic pain focuses less on modalities for pain control and more on exercises to improve strength and aerobic conditioning.

An exercise program is usually the main focus of physical therapy for people with chronic pain. A physical therapist will probably assess aerobic capacity. This often is tested in a clinic on a treadmill or bike. A home program is then established and monitored; it includes aerobic exercises, such as walking, bike riding, swimming, elliptical machines, or stairmasters. This program will gradually increase in frequency and intensity.

Along with an aerobic assessment, a physical therapist will assess a person's ability to stabilize the lumbar spine, maintain a neutral spine position, and perform abdominal bracing or hollowing. If the patient has never been to physical therapy before or is unable to perform abdominal bracing and low-level stabilization exercises, then exercises discussed in the section "Physical Therapy for Acute Pain" may be provided. The goal for a person with chronic pain, however, is to progress quickly to more dynamic stabilization and strengthening exercises that are functional and that incorporate resistance.

Dynamic stabilization involves controlling the position of the pelvis and spine during movement. People learn in therapy how to initiate and perform functional activities without pain and while dynamically stabilizing the spine in an automatic manner. A program may include higher-level stabilization exercises such as bridging (lifting the hips from the floor after bracing) with arm and leg movement and lying prone (on your stomach) with both arms and legs lifted and moving in a swimming motion. An unstable surface (Swiss ball, foam roller, or balance board) may also be incorporated into therapy to further challenge a person's ability to maintain neutral spine. Dynamic exercises will progress from the floor to sitting, kneeling, and standing positions. Eventually, people will learn how to maintain abdominal bracing and a neutral spine while performing their daily activities. For some people this may be sitting at a desk, standing for long periods, taking stairs, or doing housework. Others will learn how to remain pain-free while throwing a ball, running, jumping, playing soccer or basketball, or engaging in other forms of prolonged exercise.

An exercise program for chronic pain includes more trunk and hip strengthening exercises than a program for acute pain. An increase in muscle strength will occur as muscles are overloaded by increasing resistance or weight and repetition during exercise. Resistance can be achieved with elastic bands (commonly called *therabands*) or tubing, medicine balls, body blades, free weights, or weight machines. Moving into kneeling and standing positions increases resistance by incorporating gravity into specific stabilization exercises.

Abdominal strengthening is an important component of any chronic low back pain program. Specific exercises include curl-ups, partial sit-ups, partial sit-ups with rotation, and reverse sit-ups. Curl-ups and sit-ups can be performed on the floor or on a Swiss ball. When using a Swiss ball, a person starts by sitting on the ball and then walks their feet out until the ball is under the lower back. From this position, the person then lifts his or her upper body up toward the ceiling. Hip and knee strengthening exercises, especially in functional positions such as standing, are also usually included in an exercise program. Typically, these exercises include wall slides and sits, various types of freestanding squats, and forward and backward lunges. Resistance may be added manually by a therapist or by carrying weights or a medicine ball.

By the end of a physical therapy program, people are expected to be exercising independently at home or in a local gym or recreational center. An exercise program will include an aerobic warmup, dynamic stabilization, and strengthening exercises; trunk and hip stretching help the body cool down and help prevent injury. To relieve chronic pain and prevent a recurrence, a person must make an active and conscious lifetime commitment to exercise.

Physical Therapy for Spinal Stenosis

Spinal stenosis, a condition in which the tunnel the nerves run through becomes narrowed, is described in detail in Chapter 3. People with stenosis have difficulty standing or walking and feel better when they are sitting down. Physical therapists use these symptoms as a guide when prescribing an exercise program. Many types of interventions can be beneficial for patients with stenosis. A common exercise progression includes postural education; lower back positioning with posterior pelvic tilts; stabilization exercises targeting the abdominals and gluteals; aerobic conditioning; and stretching of the back and hip muscles (especially the muscles on the front of the leg called the hip flexors).

Aerobic conditioning initially focuses on the stationary bicycle until symptoms are decreased enough to start a gradual walking program. Extension exercises (where the body bends backward) will be avoided, and flexion exercises (where the body bends forward) will be emphasized. For example, people with stenosis will be told by therapists to avoid exercises in which they lie on their stomach, especially exercises in which they are lifting any part of their body up to the ceiling. Bridging (lying supine and lifting hips to the ceiling) is another exercise that may increase pain for some people.

Flexion exercises that are commonly prescribed for people with stenosis are performed lying on the back and sitting in a chair or on a Swiss ball. The first exercise is usually the posterior pelvic tilt. The person is instructed to lie on a flat surface and rock his pelvis back so that the lower back flattens into the ground. This movement provides more space for the nerves and usually provides temporary pain relief. Other exercises that flatten the back and help relieve pain include bringing one or both legs to the chest, performing small curl-ups or sit-ups, and rolling forward from a sitting or standing position. As a person's pain decreases, extension exercises and walking will be gradually incorporated into an exercise program in a safe and pain-free way.

Physical Therapy for Herniated Disc (Slipped Disc)

A herniated disc is when the inside of the disc escapes through the outer layer and presses on the nerves of the spine causing lower back, buttock, or leg pain. This condition is described in more detail in Chapter 3. People with herniated discs have symptoms opposite to the symptoms of people with spinal stenosis. Sitting, bending forward, and driving increase symptoms, and standing and bending backward usually relieves symptoms. As with spinal stenosis, physical therapists use these symptoms as a guide when choosing an appropriate treatment program. Many types of interventions can be beneficial for patients with herniated discs. A common exercise progression includes postural education; lower back positioning with abdominal bracing or hollowing; stabilization exercises targeting the abdominals and gluteals; aerobic conditioning; and stretching of the back and hip muscles (especially the hamstrings or the muscles at the back of the leg).

Aerobic conditioning will focus on walking or the elliptical machine. Riding a bicycle is avoided, especially at first, because sitting usually increases back or leg pain. In general, flexion exercises (where the body bends forward) will be avoided and extension exercises (where the body bends backward) will be emphasized. For example, people with a herniated disc will be told by therapists to focus on exercises where they are lying on their stomach and lifting any part of their body up to the ceiling. Exercises to avoid will usually include those requiring a sitting position and a posterior pelvic tilt. Primary goals for people with herniated discs will be to learn abdominal bracing or hollowing to maintain a neutral spine position and learning correct posture and lifting techniques.

Common extension exercises include lying on the stomach and propping on elbows or performing press-ups. In press-up exercises, the hips and legs stay on the ground and the patient uses his hands to bring the upper body up gently into extension. Hyperextension is avoided. These exercises should be pain-free or pain should centralize in the lower back if leg pain is present. Stomach exercises can progress to include arm or leg lifting and upper body lifts. The bridging exercise (lying supine and lifting hips to the ceiling) is often recommended to people with herniated disc conditions; the exercise is then progressed to incorporate arm and leg elevation. As a person's pain decreases, flexion exercises and sitting will be gradually incorporated into an exercise program in a safe and pain-free way.

Physical Therapy after Spine Surgery

A physical therapist usually visits a person in the hospital within one or two days of surgery. The primary goal is to help the patient get out of bed and walk as soon after surgery as possible. Any instructions from the surgeon about what not to do will be reviewed with the patient, and an evaluation will be performed. An evaluation will include an assessment of leg and arm range-of-motion and strength to prepare the patient to move out of the hospital bed. A physical therapist will teach the patient how to correctly move and roll in bed and to go from a lying-down position to a seated position.

After the patient sits on the edge of the bed for a while, the physical therapist will help the patient stand up and walk around the room and, if possible, down the hall. Sometimes a walker (with or without wheels) will be used to assist the patient with standing and walking; usually, a physical therapist will place a gait belt around a patient's waist for safety. A therapist holds onto the belt with one hand to help support the patient while instructing the patient on proper walking techniques. Most people hold their breath or even forget to breathe when sitting and standing for the first time after surgery. Doing so can cause excessive dizziness and increase any nausea, so the physical therapist will instruct the patient to take deep breaths and keep their chin and head up at all times. During the first visit, a person will also learn how to transfer safely from the bed to a chair and back again.

After the first visit, a physical therapist will visit the patient once or twice a day until the patient is discharged from the hospital. At each visit, the therapist will make sure the patient is walking a little farther and feels safe moving around the room. The patient will be given exercises to be performed several times a day. These exercises help increase circulation and promote healing as well as increase strength and range of motion of the truck, hip, and leg muscles. Exercises can be performed lying in bed or sitting in a chair and often include the following:

- Ankle pumps: Moving the ankles up and down and in circles in both directions to maintain muscle tone and increase leg circulation.
- Quad sets: Tightening the muscles on the top of the thigh by pushing the knees straight and holding for five to ten seconds to strengthen leg muscles.
- Hamstring sets: Pushing the heel of the foot into the bed or ground with the knee slightly bent and holding for five to ten seconds to strengthen muscles at the back of the thigh.
- Glut sets: Tightening the buttock muscles and holding for five

to ten seconds to strengthen muscles that help with standing activities.

- Short arc quads: Placing a towel roll under the knee and lifting the lower leg off a stool or the bed. The leg is held straight for five to ten seconds to strengthen muscles at the top of the thigh.
- Abdominal bracing: Tightening the muscles of the lower abdomen without moving the lower back to strengthen core muscles and promote a neutral spine position.

As a person's strength increases and pain decreases, standing exercises will be incorporated into therapy sessions. These exercises often include:

- Abdominal bracing with arms: Standing with legs bent and abdominal muscles contracted to maintain a neutral spine, raise one arm overhead and then the other. The purpose is to maintain a neutral spine while adding in the weight of the arms.
- Abdominal bracing with legs (marching or high stepping): Standing with legs bent and abdominal muscles contracted to maintain a neutral spine, raise one leg and then the other with the knee pointing toward the ceiling. Also, the person will be instructed, if possible, to kick the leg straight out in front. The purpose is to maintain a neutral spine while adding in the weight of the legs.
- Mini-squats: Slowly bending and straightening the knees to strengthen the leg muscles and maintain neutral spine position.
- Toes/heels: Pushing up onto toes and back down and then pulling toes up to the ceiling and rocking back onto heels to strengthen lower legs for walking and stairs.
- Standing abduction (side leg kicks): Standing on one leg, raise the other leg out to the side with toes pointing forward and then repeat on the other side to strengthen the side of the hip.

Before the patient is discharged from the hospital, a physical therapist will make sure that the patient has any walking assistive device, such as a walker or cane. The physical therapist will also review proper sitting, standing, and walking techniques and evaluate the patient's ability to walk up or down stairs if the person must be able to do so in order to return home. Exercises will be reviewed and the therapist will tell the patient how to increase the intensity and frequency of the exercises to continue improving strength and endurance. Most people will continue with physical therapy after they leave the hospital. Therapy can occur at home, in an outpatient clinic, or in a rehabilitation or nursing facility.

When visiting a therapist outside the hospital for the first time, it is a good idea to bring any exercise sheets and written instructions from the doctor on what to do and not to do, and tell your new therapist about any medications you are currently taking. Your physical therapist will communicate with your surgeon throughout the recovery process. Therapists and physicians work together to keep complications minimal and to speed recovery. Two to four weeks after surgery it is expected that pain will decrease and strength and endurance will improve rapidly after that for most people.

If there is any increase in redness or draining from the surgical site, increased pain, or loss of function, let your therapist know immediately and get in touch with your physician right away.

Physical therapy can help improve strength, aerobic conditioning, and posture, which help determine whether a person has chronic pain or recovers from pain and remains active and comfortable.

Eight
Making the Decision about Surgery

AN ESSENTIAL COMPONENT OF good surgical care involves helping patients set their expectations appropriately. Patients' assessment of their surgical outcome must be based on reasonable expectations of what the surgery can achieve—and what can go wrong. What do patients need to know before they opt for surgery? This chapter will endeavor to answer this essential question.

Misunderstandings about surgical outcomes—both good and bad—are common. One way to avoid misunderstandings is not to compare other people's operation with the operation you may be offered. Some surgeries have remarkably good outcomes 80 to 90 percent of the time, while other surgeries are not as routinely successful. Even the same surgery performed on two different people can result in huge improvement in one and no improvement or devastating complications and debilitation in the other. Outcomes are influenced by many factors.

Overview: Expectations and Issues

Sometimes the doctor's decision to perform surgery or the patient's decision to have surgery involves no decision at all because the surgery is absolutely necessary either to save function (and avoid paralysis) or to save the patient's life. But even in an elective operation, some people are certain they want to go ahead with surgery, either because their pain is debilitating or their function is impaired, and they aren't able to do things they want to do. Most of the time, however, the decision to have surgery is not an emergency, and that decision is a difficult one to make. A person generally reaches a decision about elective back surgery only after giving it a great deal of thought.

It's a good idea to take the time you need to decide about having surgery. Make your own decision about whether to go through with the operation once you are clear about the risks and potential benefits. Find out the chances for success with your particular operation: What is the likelihood that the operation will be successful? Find out when you could expect to see positive results: What is the timeline for recovery? What steps will you need to take to achieve success in that time frame? Before surgery you should think about what resources are available to you: What is your support network, and what will your insurance cover in terms of paying for physical therapists or visiting nurses to help you after surgery or for inpatient rehabilitation or a nursing home before you can go home?

The surgeon and your family doctor or internist must also decide whether you meet three criteria to be a candidate for surgery: First, you must have a structural problem in your back that your doctors believe is causing some or all of your symptoms. Second, your doctors must believe they can correct your problem with an operation that will relieve or substantially improve the symptoms. Third, your doctors must determine that it is medically safe for you to have the surgery.

It is important that you understand your surgeon's goals, objectives, and anticipated result of the operation and that you think it is reasonable for you to undergo the surgery. If you would only consider the operation a success if you can run a marathon, then you must discuss with your doctor about whether that is a realistic goal.

We want to emphasize this important point: As part of the decision-making process, the patient needs to state his or her expectations clearly and find out from the surgeon whether achieving these goals is likely or even possible with the proposed surgical procedure. From the surgeon's perspective, we might perceive that the patient's pain is better or resolved and that the surgery has had a successful outcome, but if the patient is dissatisfied with the results of the surgery, then the surgeon and the patient are disappointed. For example, a professional tennis player may consider the operation to be a failure if she is not able to play tennis at the same level again. Perhaps the surgeon's goal was to help the patient to play weekend tennis with relatively little pain. In this case, the difference between the patient's goal and the physician's goal would lead to disappointment for both.

Pain is a significant factor in the decision to have surgery: The patient must consider the existing back pain as well as the pain after surgery. It is impossible to convey to someone the amount of pain he or she will experience after surgery, but the memory of pain recedes. If you ask a patient in the first week after surgery whether he would have surgery again, he may say, "No way," but after a year, he would say, yes, he might do it again.

Finally, if your recovery will involve other people, you need to know who the other people will be. If you are going home but are unable to shop or dress yourself, or you will need help with the household chores, make plans ahead of time to involve those people in planning the timing of the operation and the recovery.

Questions to Ask before Surgery

When is the right time to have an operation?

For most people, back problems are a chronic condition and do not require urgent surgery. The timing of elective surgery should be based on how you feel and what impact your symptoms are having on your quality of life. Patients sometimes determine when to have surgery based on their age. They will say, "Well, I'll have it now, even though my symptoms aren't that bad, because I know it's safer to be operated on while I'm younger than when I'm older, and I just want to have it done." Or they will say, "If I'm going to have it done sometime, I may as well get it done now." However, the decision should be based on how you're feeling now and on your quality of life, not on anticipated problems down the road. The counterpoint is that there can be complications with surgery or additional symptoms may emerge because of surgery—long-term sequelae of operations may occur—and if you had delayed the surgery, you would have avoided these problems later on in your life.

That said, we can reliably predict that a number of conditions are going to worsen over time. In some situations, the window of opportunity is such that the likelihood of the patient getting better is higher the sooner we operate. This is the case with myelopathy, a compression of the spinal cord that causes symptoms in the arms and legs. Myelopathy has a history of worsening and not spontaneously improving. Taking the pressure off the spinal cord through surgery generally stops the condition from getting worse. The longer an operation is delayed, the less likely it is that the person will get better or recover any of the lost function.

If you are asking yourself whether you should get the operation done now or ten years from now, you might consider your lifestyle and your quality of life. You should go ahead with surgery whenever your lifestyle or quality of life is unacceptable. If it is unacceptable now, you shouldn't wait, and if it is acceptable and there is no pressing reason to get it done now, then wait. If you feel worse later on, you can get it done then.

Do I need to get a second opinion?

Second opinions are common, and the surgeon can help you get one. Seldom do surgeons take offense if a patient gets a second opinion. If the surgeon gets upset, then you might think about whether that surgeon is right for you. If a surgeon is that wedded to his own opinion, how well will the surgeon be able to explain things? Will the surgeon be comfortable interacting with you?

You can ask your surgeon to recommend two or three surgeons for second opinions. Then ask your internist and your friends for two or three recommendations. If the same two or three names are recommended by your surgeon, your family doctor, and your friends or relatives, then you might want to schedule visits with one or two of them.

Review your insurance plan. A second opinion may be required before surgery. Sometimes, an insurance plan will cover the cost of the second opinion if it has been requested by your internist or primary care physician.

Different surgeons may offer patients different surgical approaches: for example, surgery from the front or surgery from the back. Those differences are to some degree based on differences in the surgeon's training and experience and don't necessarily reflect a difference of opinion about the primary problem. When you get a difference of opinion, find out the extent of the difference of opinion. Is it a fundamental difference in what is wrong? One surgeon may say you have hip arthritis and another may say you have nerve pressure in your back at L1. Is there a fundamental difference in opinion in the diagnosis, or do they agree on the diagnosis and the cause of the symptoms but disagree on the approach to solve the problem?

The next questions involve considering why the surgeon has recommended this specific surgical approach. Is it based on a feeling that the results are clearly better with this specific approach, or is it that the surgeon feels more comfortable with this approach? You can ask each surgeon about his or her opinion on the other surgeon's treatment plan:

- Is it a reasonable plan but not their choice? And why?
- Or is it completely unreasonable and they would not even entertain it?
- Why is it a bad idea?
- Is it reasonable and they would be willing to do it that way?
- Is it reasonable but they would not do it that way? Why?

The points at which things can go wrong in an operation are

- the initial diagnosis of the primary problem,
- the approach taken to solving the problem,
- the execution of the surgery itself (the technical performance of the procedure),
- the recognition and treatment of complications that occur after the operation.

Sometimes the diagnosis is wrong, the operation is the wrong operation, or the patient gets a complication that is inadequately treated or wrong decisions are made about how to handle the complication—there are several ways to go down a wrong path. With some of these wrong decisions, if you subsequently do the right operation, people still get better, and the effect of the other decision-making errors are relatively minor. Other times the consequences of those decision-making errors are so major that further surgery will have little or no influence on the patient's quality of life.

What could happen to me if I have the surgery, both good and bad? And what could happen to me if I don't have the surgery, both good and bad?

For some conditions, the bad things that could happen to you if you did not have the surgery—the extremes—would be death or paralysis. The good thing that could happen to you if you had the surgery would be that your quality of life would improve. The starker the contrasts are between the bad things and good things, the easier the decision. The more nuanced the differences, the longer you should think about whether to undergo something that involves pain and suffering to get *potentially* better off than you are. You have to think about how much better off, or how much worse off, you will be in both scenarios.

Ask yourself how acceptable your current condition would be if it were permanent (that is, if you didn't have the surgery). And how likely it is that your current condition is going to improve on its own. Talk to your doctor about how long the recovery from the surgery will take because this, too, is part of the decision-making equation.

Who can I involve in the decision about surgery?

Making a decision about surgery involves input from the surgeon and everyone involved in your routine care as well from people who are specialized in the areas in which you have medical issues. Your internist, cardiologist, and other medical doctors should not necessarily be involved in the particulars of the surgery, but they should be involved in assessing the effect the surgery will have on you. An anesthesiologist and other specialists may also be involved, depending on the extent of the surgery, the risk of the surgery, and your underlying medical condition.

You have to involve your internist and any specialists, if you have them, to get their input. You are not asking them to make the decision for you but to tell you the risk of underlying medical conditions having an effect on your surgery, recovery, or final outcome. The surgeon can tell you about the undesirable results or outcomes from the surgery itself; your internist or cardiologist or other specialist can tell you the likelihood of undesirable outcomes to your overall health. If you have a poor heart, lungs, liver, or kidneys, surgery could result in permanent and irreversible negative effect (and sometimes positive effect) on those organs. It's important to know the big picture, and the big picture is something the surgeon alone can't give you, especially if you have a complicated medical history.

If you have many medical conditions, another consideration is whether your internist can be involved in your care after the operation. Does he or she have privileges at the hospital where the surgery will be performed? If not, it would be wise to have an internist, a neurologist, a cardiologist, or another specialist see you before the surgery to get to know you beforehand to familiarize themselves with your medical condition. They can participate in your medical management after surgery if necessary. That way doctors won't waste time trying to get familiar with your medical condition when you are having an acute problem that needs to be addressed immediately.

You may want to ask your surgeon to recommend other patients you can talk to who have had the same surgery. Or there may be another person working with the doctor, such as a nurse, nurse practitioner, physician's assistant, or secretary, who can give you a different perspective on length of recovery, resuming activities, and functioning on your own.

How quickly do I have to decide?

For most elective surgery, there is no need to make a decision in the surgeon's office, where very few people are able to digest all of the information they are given. Ask the surgeon if he or she can give you literature on the procedure. Take notes during your conversation with the surgeon, and bring someone else along with you when you're talking about the possibility of surgery. Bringing someone along with you gives you another person's perspective, and another person's ears and brains are working on the decision.

Some people make decisions immediately in the doctor's office, but many people are more comfortable thinking about it over a cup of coffee or dinner or even over a couple of days. Each person has his or her own method of making decisions, and you have to do what is best for you.

Should I be concerned about who my anesthesiologist is?

Suppose you have decided to have surgery. What do you need to do, if anything, about finding an anesthesiologist? If you are a healthy person, have no medical conditions that require attention, and are undergoing a straightforward operation (defined as low potential for blood loss, commonly performed, and very specific goals and objectives), you probably don't need to be too concerned about the anesthesiologist as long as he or she is someone your surgeon is comfortable with and can work with. In more complicated situations, ask your surgeon whether it matters who the anesthesiologist is, and whether the surgeon has any recommendations.

Sometimes the anesthesiologist plays a small role in the outcome of the operation, but in some complicated surgeries having an anesthesiologist who feels comfortable and experienced in such techniques as special methods of inserting a breathing tube, managing high amounts of blood loss, or a higher-than-average potential for stroke during the operation. You can ask your surgeon about the anesthesiologist's technical qualifications. Like you, they are interested in seeing you have the best outcome possible.

What does my support system look like?

You need to have a clear understanding of your social network resources (family, friends, and church support), financial resources, and insurance. After surgery, some insurance companies will pay for home care: a visiting nurse to take your vital signs and check your incision, an aide to help you with bathing and dressing, or even someone to do light housecleaning and help you with meals. Most people, however, rely on family and friends for help with the nonmedical aspects of recovery. Well before surgery you will want to talk with the people you will be relying on, whether professionals or family, to make sure they are willing and available when you need them.

Choosing a Surgeon

We talked about the doctor-patient relationship in Chapter 5. Here, we focus specifically on factors you might consider in selecting a surgeon.

First, decide what you are looking for because you need to be comfortable with your decision. *What is important to you?* For some people, bedside manner is more important than surgical skill. Some are more interested in communication skills and level of trust than in surgical skills and the surgeon's hospital affiliation. Others are primarily interested in the surgeon's level of expertise and experience. Whatever your priorities are, you need to develop a level of comfort with the surgeon.

When you talk with other people, you may hear that a particular doctor is a grumpy, gruff personality but a wonderful surgeon. You might think, "I want that person as my surgeon, not as my best friend, so that's okay." You might hear that a particular doctor may not be the most experienced surgeon but is an excellent surgeon nonetheless, a wonderful human, answers questions, and follows up after surgery. You may think, "I want that person as my surgeon

Back Pain at a Glance: What Factors Should I Consider When Selecting a Surgeon?
- Physician referrals
- Knowledge
- Surgical skill
- Bedside manner
- Approach to patient care

because someone who answers my questions makes me comfortable about my care." The decision reflects your own personality and your own style.

Another way to identify good surgeons is to find out who doctors go to for their back problems. Asking your internist or primary care provider who they would see or send a relative to for your particular problem can be an effective way of finding a good doctor.

Clearance for Surgery

Successfully going through a surgical procedure involves

- tolerating the anesthesia
- tolerating the surgical procedure (being able to tolerate the stress that is placed on the body as a result of the surgery)
- tolerating blood loss and possibly blood replacement
- tolerating various drugs that are administered during anesthesia and surgery
- getting through the critical postoperative period
- healing from the surgery, which includes the healing of soft tissues and, if the goal of the operation was fusion, the healing of bones properly
- regaining your strength and maximizing your function after surgery

Contact your medical doctor, and make sure he or she knows you are having an operation. Usually, the patient's family physician or internist assesses the patient medically before surgery, including a physical examination and functional tests of the body's various systems. Some of the systems can be assessed simply by ordering a blood test. Others may require more advanced tests, and different levels of testing may be necessary for different patients.

Blood work ordered by the physician includes studies to assess the function of these organs and to look at the patient's coagulation capacity (whether the blood is clotting normally). If someone has a blood-clotting problem, either as a result of medications or because of a blood disease, then that would pose a significant risk of blood clots during the surgery as well as immediately after the operation. The coagulation capacity is fully assessed and if necessary corrected before surgery.

For a young person with no history of cardiac problems, extensive cardiac testing might be unnecessary, whereas an older person with known heart risks or heart disease may require one or more tests to assess heart function and cardiac risk before surgery.

To find out whether the heart can withstand surgery, two tests may be performed: (1) an electrocardiogram (EKG), which is the test where wires and pads are attached to your body and the electrical activity of the heart is recorded, and (2) an echocardiogram (echo), which looks at the heart using a sonar (ultrasound) device to see how well the heart is contracting. Sometimes more extensive studies may be necessary, such as a cardiac stress test and cardiac catheterization.

Back Pain at a Glance: Which Body Systems Are Assessed before Surgery?

- The cardiovascular system: the heart and the blood vessels
- The pulmonary system: the lungs and breathing capacity
- The liver (whether the liver is functioning adequately to metabolize all the drugs given during the operation)
- The kidneys

Informed Consent

The consent process is a discussion between you and the surgeon about the nature of your problem, his or her approach for addressing that problem, and the *relative* risks and benefits and *expected* risks and benefits of the surgery and alternative forms of treatment. This discussion takes place before you sign a permission form for the surgery. (Relative risk and expected risk are concepts addressed earlier in this chapter.) This discussion is important and ends in the signing of a document by you giving the surgeon permission to perform the surgery. The discussion and consent signing often take place in the doctor's office in advance of the day of surgery.

Nine
Back Surgery and Recovery

IF YOU ARE SCHEDULED for surgery, this means that you and your surgeon have taken steps to arrive at the decision to proceed with surgery. First, your surgeon believes that there is a high likelihood that the cause of your problem has been identified. Second, the surgeon believes that you are likely to benefit from surgery; for example, surgery will likely bring some relief from pain and restore some function, but it may not resolve all of your problems. The surgeon may have done additional tests to clarify the surgical plan. Finally, you have been medically assessed by your physician, and, in your physician's opinion, you can safely be put under anesthesia and you have the capacity to heal from the surgery.

If you know that you are going to have a surgical procedure, one of the best things you can do is take care of you. Eat nutritional, well-balanced meals, get plenty of sleep, exercise within your limits (keep moving if possible, and as your doctor advises you), stop smoking, and limit or eliminate alcoholic beverages. You want to be in top physical and emotional shape when the day of surgery arrives.

In an emergency, of course, there is no time to think about whether to have the surgery and no time to build up your physical reserve. Surgical procedures on the back require general anesthesia, so we begin this chapter with a discussion of anesthesia.

Preparing for Surgery

Anesthesia

General anesthesia poses certain risks. Before surgery, we must be sure that a person is in good physical shape to withstand the anesthesia. To assess a person's fitness for anesthesia, we check whether the patient has any previously undetected significant medical conditions that might pose a problem during anesthesia or immediately after the surgery. Individuals with cardiac disease are more prone to heart attacks. Patients with liver or kidney problems may see these conditions worsen after surgery. We also are concerned about the possibility of strokes, seizures, and allergic reactions to medications used in anesthesia and to other medications.

The anesthesiologist plays a critical role in making the final decision about whether the patient can be placed under anesthesia. For example, the anesthesiologist assesses whether a breathing tube can be easily placed in the patient. If this is going to be a difficult procedure, the anesthesiologist can take special precautions to address problems that may arise. The anesthesiologist's assessment of the patient can be very extensive. In most instances it is straightforward and involves a history, physical examination, a review of laboratory values, an EKG, and a chest radiograph.

Blood Banking

Most of the time surgeons are operating because of specific problems, and they are trying to achieve specific goals and objectives. Moreover, most of the time they know, from experience, approximately how much blood the patient will lose, within a reasonable range.

Although the supply of donated blood in this country is safe, many people are concerned about receiving transfusions of donated blood as part of an operation, and they ask about donating their own blood (called *autologous blood banking*) before the surgery.

The amount of blood that is lost in a spine operation ranges from a thimbleful to many gallons—even more blood than your body holds at one time.

When you get right down to it, few people really should give blood for spine operations. Autologous blood banking is not needed and is not a good idea for smaller operations such as lumbar discectomy or cervical fusions in which very little blood is lost during the operation. Autologous blood banking is also not needed for larger operations because so much blood is lost that you will not be able to give enough blood in advance to replace it. If you are going to be losing less than the equivalent of two pints of blood, you don't need to bank blood, and if you are going to be losing more than four pints of blood, you probably don't need to bank blood. If you are over age 70, it is not a good idea to give your own blood. If you have heart conditions or other conditions such as anemia that would make it risky for you to give blood, you shouldn't give blood. For prostate surgery and joint replacement surgery, autologous blood banking often makes more sense that it does for spine surgery.

If you *are* going to donate autologous blood, it needs to be planned for and donated at least several weeks before the operation. You have to give your blood a number of weeks in advance because the blood needs to be processed and tested, and that processing does not happen overnight. There also has to be enough time for your body to compensate for some of the blood that you gave. *The general rule is one week per pint donated.* Finally, if you are going to donate autologous blood, keep yourself well hydrated before and after the blood is taken.

When someone does not donate blood in advance or needs more blood than has been donated a variety of methods are available to provide adequate replacement blood.

Donor blood from a blood bank that matches the patient's own blood type can be used. Another method used is to collect, clean, and reuse patients' own blood lost during the course of surgery. This is called *cell saver blood.* This blood is collected through a special suctioning device; tissue and other material that is being suctioned can be separated from the blood. A processing machine cleans the blood and puts it through a filter, and the blood is then returned to the person as a blood transfusion. This process allows us to capture some of the patient's own blood that is lost in the operation and give it back to the patient.

Medications

It is important for patients to tell their doctor *all* the medications they are taking, both medications prescribed by a physician (prescription drugs) and over-the-counter (OTC) medications. The doctor *must* be told whether you are taking blood thinners such as aspirin, Coumadin, or heparin. Blood thinners are prescribed by the physician when a patient has a blood clot, certain heart conditions, or a history of stroke or cardiac irregularities. The effects of these medications can be long-lasting, such as aspirin, for example, which is a potent blood thinner. Stopping the aspirin the day before the operation does not allow the body enough time to resume the normal clotting mechanism. It has to be taken out of the system for *at least five to seven days* before the surgical procedure.

In emergency circumstances, we accept the risk involved in operating on someone who is taking blood thinners, and we take corrective actions before and during the operating room to help us deal with that problem, but for elective cases, there is no reason to take that kind of risk. Tell your surgeon about any blood thinners you are taking well before the day of surgery.

The Day before Surgery

Usually the patient does not come into the hospital the day before surgery, but the patient is asked to follow our instructions at home on that day. We instruct the patient not to eat or drink anything after midnight. This is very important because it helps reduce the risk of aspiration during induction of anesthesia. The lung injury that could occur can lead to pneumonia. Clearly, lung aspiration of stomach contents can be a serious problem, so it is important: *Do not eat or drink anything after midnight.*

The night before surgery you can take many of your regular medications. If you are taking the medications more often than every eight hours, the anesthesiologist usually will tell you whether to take specific medications the night before surgery or the morning of surgery, usually with a small sip of water to push the medications down. It is better not to put anything in the stomach before surgery, however. Again, in emergency circumstances, we sometimes have to accept the risk and perform an operation on someone who has recently eaten, but for elective operations, ideally, the patient's stomach will be empty for about eight hours before surgery.

The Surgery

When you arrive at the hospital on the morning of the operation, first you will meet with the anesthesiologist, who will look through your records, ask about your medications, making sure you have stopped all the medications that could be a problem during surgery. The anesthesiologist will look at your airway, checking, again, to see how a breathing tube can be placed safely.

You will also see a nurse who will ask you to verify that you are having the specific procedure for which you signed the consent form (see Chapter 8). If you are going to have a back operation and the nurse tells you that you are scheduled for a different operation than you are expecting to undergo such as a knee surgery when you expect to be undergoing a spine operation, you need to speak up. Verify with the nurse that you're having the correct surgery. Ask to speak to your surgeon if you have any concerns about the procedure to be performed. Before surgery the surgeon (or a member of the surgical team) will write his or her initials on the site of the surgery.

Once you are put to sleep, you are positioned to give the surgeon access to the part of the spine to be operated on. The back or neck is cleaned, prepared, and draped.

Before the operation starts, there is a "time out," wherein everyone stops, the surgeon states the patient's name (identifies the patient), and announces the type of surgery to be performed. Everyone in the operating room has to agree that the correct patient is there and that the patient is having the operation stated on the consent form. Everyone agrees on the operation that is about to take place. Once the surgeon, the nurse, and the anesthesiologist agree that they have identified the patient and that they are clear about what's going to be done, then the operation can proceed.

X-rays and imaging studies are displayed in the operating room to orient the surgeon; these images identify the pathology and the focus of the operation and assist the surgeon during the operation. The surgeon can also obtain different types of imaging during the operation: plain x-rays, fluoroscopy (which provides "live" pictures of the spine), and computer-assisted image guidance or navigation, which is calibrated to preoperative CT (computed tomography) scans and MRIs (magnetic resonance imaging).

Many things are done during the operation, including giving the patient antibiotics and fluids. Techniques are employed that minimize blood loss and pain, such as infiltrating epinephrine (which constricts blood vessels) into the soft tissues to reduce the amount of bleeding, using local anesthetics such as lidocaine before skin incisions, and putting medications into the sac around the spinal cord to minimize postoperative pain.

Studies have shown that the use of local anesthetics during surgery decreases the overall use of pain medications during the patient's hospitalization. The local anesthetics block stimulation of the pain response, thereby blocking pain before it gets started. The anesthesiologist can do other things to block the stimulation of the pain response. Right before the end of surgery, for example, the patient can be given narcotics directly into the spinal canal, bathing the spinal nerves to try to decrease pain after surgery. These methods have varying degrees of success, depending on which approach is used and how the patient responds to them.

Sometimes events occur, but they are not recognized during the operation, and people wake up having had a stroke or having had a heart attack. Because the patient is monitored closely during surgery, you might expect that heart attacks would always be recognized by the medical professionals in the operating room. However, the monitoring equipment monitors the rate and the rhythm of the heart rather than the often subtle changes associated with heart attacks. If a heart attack or stroke is recognized during surgery, the procedure is in most cases altered or stopped.

After Surgery

The patient is awakened in the operating room by the anesthesia team and asked to move his or her arms and legs before leaving the

OR. Depending on the magnitude of the surgery and the medical condition of the patient, the patient is transferred either to an intensive care unit or the recovery room. In the immediate postoperative period, patients are checked to ensure that they are breathing comfortably on their own, their blood pressure is stable, pain is minimized, and blood and fluids are adequately replaced.

If the patient is healthy and the surgery does not mandate an intensive care unit bed after surgery, the patient is taken to the recovery room for several hours. After the recovery room, the patient is moved to a hospital room for the remainder of the hospital stay. Some patients need to be in the intensive care unit—for example, if we need to monitor or support the patient's breathing, blood pressure, or both more closely after the operation. The breathing tube may be left in for several hours or several days after the surgery, depending on the patient's medical condition and the type of surgery. Drains are often placed in the surgical site to drain the blood and fluid and a catheter in the urethra drains urine and empties the bladder. The drains and catheter are removed over the course of the patient's hospital stay.

A variety of postoperative pain medications are used to treat pain during the recovery period. Usually before you can eat, you are given an IV with a button you can push to receive pain medicine from a computer-activated pump. We often use narcotic medications that are inserted directly into the bloodstream through an IV with a pump that you control. After the first, second, or third day, depending on the extent of the operation, patients are switched to an oral pain reliever. Intravenous pain medications are stronger and more effective than pills, but their effects last for a short time. Pills, however, require your stomach to be functioning so you can absorb the medication. The need for pain medication gradually decreases as the days progress.

For a few hours to several days after surgery, you may have a condition called an *ileus*. An ileus is when your stomach and intestines stop functioning, and there is a build-up of fluids. The more extensive the operation, the more likely it is that an ileus will occur. You can't eat or drink anything because it would just fill up your stomach and make you nauseous and vomit. Your stomach may be distended. An ileus is treated by minimizing the use of any medications that are contributing to the problem (recall that narcotics can be constipating) and sometimes by stimulating a bowel movement with a laxative or other medication. The patient is fed and hydrated through IV catheters until the stomach and intestines recover.

The dura is the covering around the spinal cord and spinal nerves and contains the spinal fluid. When we do a surgical procedure in which we open the dura and enter the spinal fluid space, such as for a tumor, we close the covering as best we can with sutures and tissue patches. However, we cannot do as good a job as the body can, so we generally keep the patient flat for twenty-four to seventy-two hours, until the dura seals, and then we sit the patient up and get the patient out of bed. If the patient is allowed to sit up too soon, spinal fluid can leak, and a severe headache from that leakage can occur.

In most instances, getting up as soon as possible after an operation is important to the recovery process. Often your doctor will want you to be up, walking, and moving around within one or two days after an operation. Patients are encouraged to walk, usually with the help of a physical therapist. It's uncomfortable, but it's important. It improves the circulation in your legs and helps prevent blood clots, pneumonia, and other fatal conditions that could occur after the operation. In most instances, pressure stockings, such as compressible air stockings, are placed on the patient's legs, and some patients are given heparin subcutaneously (injected under the skin) after major surgery to prevent blood clots.

Leaving the Hospital

A patient is ready to leave the hospital when body functions are normal, pain is controlled, and activity has increased to an acceptable level to function at home. Before being discharged, the patient will receive discharge instructions explaining what they can and cannot do, how to care for the wound, when to return for follow-up evaluation, and whether x-ray studies need to be performed before the patient's next doctor's visit. The patient will receive a list of symptoms to watch for, such as:

- Redness or draining (which may be signs of infection)
- Fever
- Increased pain
- Loss of function

If you have any of these symptoms, you need to get in touch with your physician right away.
Rather than going home, some people go to a rehabilitation center or nursing home, depending on their physical capacity to exercise. Someone who is capable of doing physical therapy for several hours a day often will go to a rehabilitation hospital, where the focus is to try to improve physical capacity so they can be independent at home. Over the course of a week or three weeks, we expect that the patient's physical capacity will rapidly improve. Someone who has limited potential to improve her physical capacity over time will often go to a skilled nursing facility or a subacute rehabilitation center, where the focus is not on physical rehabilitation but on providing physical support while the patient regains strength.

Postsurgery Complications

Once you leave the hospital, it's important to know what to look for and how to contact people day, night, and on weekends. Keep a list of phone numbers nearby so you know you will be able to reach someone at all times because complications can occur even in a normal course of recovery. The following complications, while not likely, are possible:

- Wound complications, including infection or lack of healing.
- After-surgery pneumonia.
- After-surgery blood clots that can travel from your legs into your lungs.
- Hardware complications, including malposition of the hardware (putting the hardware in the wrong position), migration of the hardware into the wrong position, or loosening of the hardware.
- For a fusion procedure, bones not growing together (which is a

nonunion) or growing together in the wrong position (which is a malunion).

- Nerve complications, including pressure on the nerves from fluid (such as blood or cerebral spinal fluid or serum), hardware, or bone.
- New fractures in the bones.

The time line for complications is relatively predictable. The things that happen earliest are wound complications such as a seroma, which is fluid accumulation under the skin or under the soft tissue and a blood clot in the legs, called a *deep vein thrombosis* (DVT). A DVT is painful and can dislodge from the leg, move up to the lungs (*pulmonary emboli*), and could lead to death. Avoiding a DVT is one reason to get up and move around as soon as possible: The earlier you move around and the more active you are, the less likely you will to develop a DVT. After surgery, a patient may develop pneumonia from having had general anesthesia and from lying in bed, not expanding lungs to their full volume.

The next complications would be infections or the wound not healing.

Antibiotics are given before surgery and for twenty-four hours after surgery, but infections can develop at any time. When you are discharged, you will have a list of the warning signs of infection and a list of people to contact if you develop an infection (or any other complication). If an infection develops, surgery and/or antibiotics are used to treat the infection. A drain may be put in the wound, which may require another operation to clean out the wound. When the wound opens up without an infection, in what is called a dehiscence, it may be necessary to clean out the wound and reclose the incision using different techniques, followed sometimes by a short course of antibiotics.

The complications that occur later in the postsurgery process include hardware complications such as loosening or migration of hardware. Even later complications include nonunion, when the bones don't heal.

A theme in our surgical practice, and the theme of this book, is that back surgery is not surgery to be undertaken until the patient and the physician have given serious thought to the need for the surgery, the patient's expectations for the results of the surgery, and the patient's ability to safely undergo and recover from surgery. When surgery is necessary and the patient and his or her physicians decide to proceed, then there are procedures and precautions in place (many of them described in this chapter) to make the surgery as safe and as successful as possible.

Index